# HEALTHY HAPPY ADHD

# HEALTHY HAPPY ADHD

TRANSFORM HOW YOU MOVE,
EAT, AND FEEL, AND CREATE
YOUR OWN PATH TO
WELL-BEING

## Lisa Dee

RODALE
New York

A Rodale Trade Paperback Original

Published in the United States by Rodale Books, an imprint of Random House, a division of Penguin Random House LLC, 1745 Broadway, New York, NY, 10019.

Rodale & Plant with colophon is a registered trademark of Penguin Random House LLC.

LIBRARY OF CONGRESS CATALOGING-IN-PUBLICATION DATA
Names: Dee, Lisa, author.
Title: Healthy happy ADHD / Lisa Dee.
Description: First paperback edition. | New York, NY: Rodale, [2025] | Includes bibliographical references and index.
Identifiers: LCCN 2024035577 (print) | LCCN 2024035578 (ebook) | ISBN 9780593797020 (trade paperback) | ISBN 9780593797037 (ebook)
Subjects: LCSH: People with attention-deficit hyperactivity disorder—Life skills guides. | Attention-deficit hyperactivity disorder in adults.
Classification: LCC RC394.A85 D445 2025 (print) | LCC RC394.A85 (ebook) | DDC 616.85/89—dc23/eng/20241010
LC record available at https://lccn.loc.gov/2024035577
LC ebook record available at https://lccn.loc.gov/2024035578

Printed in the United States of America on acid-free paper

RodaleBooks.com | RandomHouseBooks.com
penguinrandomhouse.com

1st Printing

Book design by Jo Anne Metsch

The authorized representative in the EU for product safety and compliance is Penguin Random House Ireland, Morrison Chambers, 32 Nassau Street, Dublin D02 YH68, Ireland, https://eu-contact.penguin.ie.

To the hopeful girl in us all

# Contents

# Introduction

"I can't stick to anything."

This is a sentence I've heard countless times over the last decade while working with women as a health and fitness coach. As if sticking to a to-do list, the same gym regimen, hobby, diet, or calorie count *forever* is the ultimate achievement.

If you're reading this book, I'm going to guess that you're one of the ADHD women in the world who *want* to feel better. You desire a deeper level of health and happiness in your life. You crave a feeling of calm in your life. You're totally over jumping from journal to journal, diet to diet, expecting each new thing to be the secret to changing how you see yourself, and how you approach your habits and lifestyle. You just want to feel healthy, happy, in love with your life.

That was definitely my experience many times during my life, especially in 2021. I had impulsively taken on law school while also running my coaching business. A truckload of trauma from the past was surfacing and I was in therapy, which resulted in a post-traumatic stress disorder (PTSD) diagnosis. A long stint of comfort eating had had me slowly gaining weight over the two previous years. I was over-whelmed and deeply struggling.

I had worked with women for eight years to help them build habits that supported their bodies, minds, and spirits. I guided many, many transformations over that time. Yet here I was feeling unhealthy, unfit, and unhappy. I was slow and heavy on my feet and got out of breath while climbing the stairs. A zeal for life, a love for progress, a passion for fitness, an optimistic outlook, and a playful excitement for making my dreams a reality were core elements of who I was. But I didn't see myself that way anymore. My entire self-concept had changed. I began to believe that I was someone who was too lazy to go for a walk, who couldn't be bothered to eat healthy, and who opted to sit around feeling sorry for herself instead of taking responsibility for what she *could* change.

I couldn't seem to fully admit that I was struggling because that brought a feeling of deep shame. So I pretended I was fine and did what I knew best: I put on a brave face for the world. I had stopped living by my values and ethos, so much so that people stopped asking me for advice about their well-being. This lack of vibrancy flowed into all areas of my life. At first I felt dissatisfied and frustrated, but soon I began to feel helpless, hopeless, and *empty*.

One night, I was crouched over my desk in my kitchen, struggling with two deadlines that fell in the same week. My accountant had asked me to input some transactions into their system so they could file my paperwork on time, avoiding a penalty. At the same time, a deadline for a short essay for one of my law classes was looming. I had left both the tax return and the essay until the last moment, and I couldn't seem to work on either task for more than a few minutes at a time.

My brain was going a million miles an hour, and I kept erupting into floods of tears. On paper, both tasks seemed quite simple and normal entries on any functioning adult's daily to-do list.

*Why can't I just do them?* I asked myself.

*It's not even hard, so why can't I just do it?*

*What's wrong with me?*

*This is so easy for other people.*

*Every single month, I make this same mistake.*

*If I can't do even these two simple things, how am I EVER going to be able to do bigger things in life?*

*I'll never be able to take care of children.*

*I'm such a mess.*

*They think I'm lazy.*

*I'm capable of better.*

I felt embarrassed. I felt stupid. I felt like I was going backward in life. I hated myself at that moment. I knew it wasn't "normal" for a woman in her thirties to struggle like this so often. There were women juggling way bigger responsibilities than mine, and they seemed fine. This kind of situation replayed itself many times during that year of my life. I would sit in law school classes, bored out of my mind from the lack of stimulation. I was distracted, daydreaming, wishing I could be anywhere else. At the same time, I wanted to get the degree and save the world. I would kick myself during exam time because I knew the content. It wasn't hard to understand, but it was hard to remember and implement the information in the essays and assignments. One excited angel on one shoulder was telling me all I was capable of and the potential I had yet to tap into, while on the other shoulder was a gremlin who reminded me of all the ways I was behind and "less than."

After many more inexplicable meltdowns at my desk, an Instagram post about ADHD caught my attention. Recognizing myself in the description and needing to know more, I searched for podcasts on ADHD. I listened to a few episodes in a row while I was on a walk, and I couldn't get enough. I felt so seen. Learning that someone with ADHD has an interest-driven nervous system instead of an importance-driven nervous system explained why I so often avoided doing the mundane, everyday tasks that most adults seem to have no problem doing, such as completing paperwork and following through on long-term projects. I often found it challenging to stay on top of household chores and bills, but I could spend hours engrossed in a creative project without even realizing the passing of time. I was so fired up that I ran all the way home and burst through the door to tell my partner, Ruairí, "*I think I have ADHD.*"

I went down a research rabbit hole, reading and listening to everything about how ADHD affects women. Suddenly, so much made sense, such as the way my body constantly felt like it was jumping out of itself. I was always changing positions, putting my hair behind my ear every few minutes even when there was no hair to move, sipping my drink, scribbling, flicking my pen, fixing my socks, picking my nails, darting my eyes around every room. Until learning about ADHD, I'd never thought much about this constant fidgeting and activity. It was just the way I was. Now I knew it was hyperactivity from my ADHD. I felt so relieved that I cried. I knew I had found something important that explained a lifetime of patterns that I hadn't understood before. Deep down, I knew this was a missing piece of the puzzle.

I had already seen both a therapist and then a clinical psychologist the year before who had diagnosed me with PTSD, but to find out if I had ADHD, I needed to go to a psychiatrist. I searched for one who specialized in ADHD and found someone who could see me a few weeks later.[*]

I was late to my appointment. I tried to be polite, smiley, and optimistic and held back on telling him how bad I felt at times. I was embarrassed about the seemingly basic tasks I would cry about and didn't want this professional to judge me.[†]

My mask didn't work, and thirty minutes later, he told me I have severe ADHD. The psychiatrist gave me a prescription for medication, but I wasn't sure about starting it. I saw medication as a life-changing decision and worried I would get hooked or so dependent on it that I wouldn't be able to stop taking it. He assured me that this was unlikely and that ADHD medication was transformative for so many women like me, but I still didn't feel comfortable with it, especially when I hadn't addressed my lifestyle choices first. I wanted to feel as good as I could so that if I ever decided to take

---

[*] I live in the United Kingdom. Wait times for evaluations weren't so long back then, but I understand that at the time of this writing in 2023, they are a minimum of six months at the National Health Service and with many private providers. Wait times vary widely depending on location and country. ADHD can be officially diagnosed by specialist psychiatrists, but options and diagnostic criteria may differ in other countries. My hope is that timely support will soon become available for women with undiagnosed ADHD. The number of women who need support is heartbreaking.

[†] Don't do what I did. Let it all out. Don't hold back. You're literally paying someone to help you the best they can, and they can't help you if you're not sharing your experiences for fear of being judged, rejected, or laughed at.

meds, I could see the difference they made from a new baseline instead of from my vantage point at the time — physically, mentally, and emotionally unwell.

I knew that helping me carry out lifestyle changes wasn't the psychiatrist's job; I needed to figure out this piece of the puzzle for myself and play a part in my own story of healing. I decided to take things into my own hands and go back to basic healthy-living practices, enlisting help where needed. I found ways to better manage my everyday life, to feel better, and to drop the excess weight I was carrying. This work gave me direction—something positive to focus on.

In the coming chapters, I'll share the thoughts, ideas, and habits that I feel truly transformed me after my ADHD diagnosis, along with many other practices I have added over time. Just a few months after my diagnosis, I no longer felt like the desperate, powerless girl who showed up in front of the psychiatrist that day. Two years later, I still haven't needed to go on meds for ADHD. I try to live by these habits and practices I'll relate to you as best I can. I don't do them perfectly or 100 percent of the time, but I take a good, honest shot at taking care of myself, because when I don't, ADHD rules my life.

When I am following my Healthy Happy ADHD habits and practices, my ADHD symptoms feel less intense. I have more energy and mental clarity, I'm in a better mood, and I can focus more deeply. If I have a bad day, week, or month (which happens), I'm aware of the thoughts and practices I need to return to that help me feel good again. I've developed a deeper and more compassionate relationship with myself. I don't beat myself up as often for not being like everyone else. I'm careful about the people I allow in my life. I feel better in my body. I've learned to live in tune with its natural rhythms, helping it return to a more vibrant state. I now appreciate how the body responds when we come at it from a place of love and care instead of disgust and hate.

To live the life you wish to live—one full of energy, creativity, love, flow, excitement, success, and the freedom just to be yourself—you must take care of your foundation. The eight core pillars that I'll focus on in the book will help you connect with yourself, get to know who you are, release shame, and nourish your body and mind. They'll show you how to experience the best of who you are while reducing and better managing the not-so-enjoyable ADHD traits that can make living almost impossible. They'll help you feel your best on the inside so you can go into the outside world and dazzle, as you were always meant to. They'll give your life more structure specifically around health and wellness, which will lift your mood, energy, focus, fitness, health, and happiness. I felt compelled to write this book for women who need somewhere to turn for lifestyle support for their ADHD, whether they already have a diagnosis or are waiting for an evaluation. As far as I know, there isn't any other book like this out there.

It's what I wish I had had when I first thought I might have ADHD—a book that focuses on health, fitness, and well-being for women with ADHD *by* a woman with ADHD. A book that closes the gap between a clinical approach and lived experience and shows women they really can have ADHD *and* become healthy and happy.

---

*To live the life you wish to live—one full of energy, creativity, love, flow, excitement, success, and the freedom just to be yourself—you must take care of your foundation.*

---

Living with ADHD can be debilitating, excruciating, and overwhelming, but it can also be beautiful, adventurous, fulfilling, and freeing if you can find ways to let it be. With the right outlook on life and tailored habits to support you, you can finally step into being the superstar you are. You can pump rocket fuel into all the ADHD traits that make you great: your creativity, your ability to focus on what excites you in your soul, your compassion and ability to deeply connect with and see others, your out-of-the-box thinking and natural problem-solving skills (an incredible asset to any company, organization, or community that you're a part of, or create!), your natural drive toward entrepreneurialism, your talent for leading a group of people to a greater good and a more efficient way of working in this world.

This doesn't mean that your ADHD will magically go away. If you've picked up this book in the hope it will help you *fit in* with the world around you, put it back down. You're not broken, or in need of fixing or changing to fit in with the world. You've just forgotten who you are as you've struggled to keep up with the world around you—and it's making you feel deeply unwell. ADHD makes a lot of things harder, but it doesn't have to be a life sentence of pain, and that is the hill I choose to die on. You can make a lot of lifestyle shifts to manage your ADHD differently and feel better. You can rearrange your life, your thoughts, and your beliefs to work *with* your ADHD instead of against it.

**As you read this book, I want you to take what you need and leave the rest.** There's no such thing as a one-size-fits-all approach to ADHD. Just because you and I both have ADHD doesn't mean our experiences will be the same. I present the chapter pillars in the order that I discovered them and incorporated them into my life, but I encourage you to use the information in the way that works best for you. Some teachings will resonate with you while others won't. You might find something new each time you revisit the book. You might read the book from beginning to end. Or, when reading feels hard, you might just flip through the pages and read the bolded lines, quotes, and headings that jump out at you. (You'll still get a sense of the most important ideas if you do.) Trust your instincts, make choices that resonate with you, and embrace being your own guide. Don't wait for science or anyone else to dictate how you should live. There are things science has yet to study, and that may not happen in your lifetime. It's your life to lead. You are your own guru, and underneath the overwhelm, you intuitively know what feels right for you.

---

*You are your own guru, and underneath the overwhelm, you intuitively know what feels right for you.*

---

I hope this book helps you reconnect with your most vibrant self. I hope it guides you to what feels right and gives you the confidence to choose it. I hope you feel curious and courageous enough to explore new thoughts, ideas, and lifestyle practices. I hope you see yourself differently.

It's time for transformation.

It's time to let go of shame.

It's time to come back to who you are.

We need to break the vicious cycle that repeats itself.

We need to clear out the old to make space for the new.

You'll no longer tolerate being pressured to hide who you are.

The small stuff won't get to you as much or as often as it used to.

Hard days will still come, but you'll be better equipped to deal with them.

You'll feel free, energetic, magnetic, and beautiful, infusing joy into all you do.

A whole new way of being is awaiting you.

# HEALTHY HAPPY ADHD

# 1

##### ■

# Change How You See ADHD

*Break the cycle and create a new story.*

While ADHD affects every woman differently, one thing remains true for us all: An unhealthy lifestyle can make the negative parts of ADHD more intense. And let's face it, when these negative parts include distractibility, disorganization, emotional dysregulation, anxiety, and executive dysfunction, life as an adult in this world is inevitably going to be more challenging and less enjoyable.

You deserve to live a life of joy, fulfillment, health, vibrancy, and happiness. You deserve to feel healthy and happy. There are practices you can bring into your life to improve how you feel, and these practices will help protect you from future overwhelm and burnout.

## ADHD TRAPS YOU IN A VICIOUS CYCLE

There are many reasons why our ADHD struggles get in the way of leading a healthy lifestyle. Here are the most common ways that they can keep us from maintaining good habits like regular exercise. You're probably already familiar with some of them.

- **Boredom intolerance:** Traditional workouts might not hold your attention for long, and repetitive exercises can feel tedious. You get bored with workout routines easily and think there's no point in making one if you can't stick to it. When you do start a new routine, you eventually stop, give up, and call it another failure.

- **Difficulties with time management:** You feel like you have all the time in the world and that you can just do it later, but "later" never comes. Or you feel you have no time to do anything because you have an appointment at 3:00 p.m. and therefore can only sit and wait for said appointment so you won't miss it.

- **Executive dysfunction:** "Executive dysfunction" is a term that describes having difficulties with organizing, planning, initiating, completing, and switching between tasks. For example, you might have trouble sticking to a plan and prioritizing a goal. You want to go to the gym, but on your drive there, you feel sleepy, so you stop at a café to grab a coffee. You realize you need to pee, and this reminds you that you need to pick up toilet paper at the store. You stop by the store to get it, and suddenly, before you know it, you're doing a full grocery shopping run, only to see the time and realize three hours have passed and you can't go to the gym because you need to be home in time to take an important work call.

- **Emotional dysregulation:** When you have ADHD, you don't feel just a little bit; you feel everything a lot. Emotional dysregulation means you have trouble calming down once you're upset or you have massive reactions to objectively small issues. Someone cutting in front of you in traffic could be the last straw to bring you to tears. You know you're not crying over the person cutting in front of you. As your body floods with emotion, you might not be able to process how you're feeling or you react impulsively. Fluctuating emotions can drain energy and motivation, making it hard to find the drive to maintain a healthful habit, even if you intellectually understand its benefits.

- **Overwhelm:** When stress and the demands of everyday life pile up, your brain has trouble filtering and sorting all the incoming data from the world around you. There are looming deadlines, unfinished projects, dirty clothes scattered everywhere, unread emails building up, and late payment reminders. Eventually, if you're at full capacity, you might enter a state of shutdown. You might find it hard to speak or move, let alone sign up for a yoga class or prepare a healthy meal. You might feel a sense of powerlessness over your body and your life.

- **Anxiety:** If you're always late to class or work, forgetting important tasks, feeling disorganized and leaving projects until the last minute, and afraid of getting in trouble, of course you're feeling anxious! Anxiety-driven perfectionism can make you hesitant to try something new, such as starting to exercise or a new workout, if you fear not being able to achieve your goals perfectly. Over time, it can affect your confidence, self-esteem, and self-worth, and eventually lead to burnout and health problems.

- **Negative self-image:** You see yourself as lazy, a hot mess who can never stick to anything and isn't able to change. You would never bother going to the gym because, why? As far as you can tell, this "lazy mess" is *who you are* and nothing will ever change that. Your negative self-concept is so embedded in you after years of reinforcement that it's become your identity, making change difficult. (We'll discuss why the way we see ourselves is so important in chapter 3.)

- **Unhelpful coping mechanisms:** When faced with painful emotions or stress, you might turn to coping mechanisms to self-soothe. You might self-medicate with substances like alcohol, procrastinate on a task to avoid the discomfort associated with it (yes, procrastination is a coping mechanism!), or turn to sugary foods for comfort. These coping mechanisms provide a quick escape from pain and the pressures of daily life, but they can exacerbate ADHD symptoms, worsen mood swings, and breed more unhealthy habits.

**Because you have ADHD, it's hard to have a healthy lifestyle, but *not* having a healthy lifestyle makes ADHD worse. This creates a vicious cycle that leaves many of us with ADHD feeling helpless and prevents us from experiencing true health and happiness.**

This cycle can continue into infinity. As it repeats, we can begin believing that we're stuck in a world where nothing seems to change for the better. We might find ourselves feeling powerless. We repeatedly tell ourselves that there's nothing we can do to break the cycle, that the world just wasn't built for us and because of that, we're doomed to a lifetime of unhappiness. If we live too many days looking through *this* lens, it can become our outlook on life. Resigning ourselves to thinking *this is just how it is* can lead us to feel hopeless and to

## THE VICIOUS CYCLE

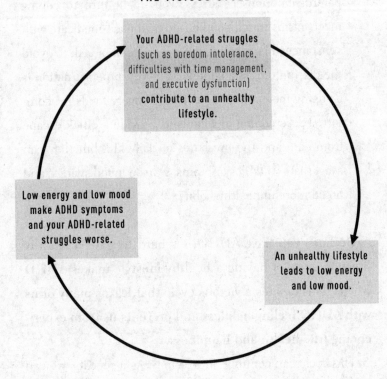

Your ADHD-related struggles (such as boredom intolerance, difficulties with time management, and executive dysfunction) **contribute to an unhealthy lifestyle.**

**An unhealthy lifestyle leads to low energy and low mood.**

Low energy and low mood make ADHD symptoms and your ADHD-related struggles worse.

neglect self-care and self-love. We can end up deeply depressed and sliding down a slope of blame, pain, and shame. I've argued for my limitations and held tightly to problems, using them as evidence of my helplessness. It felt comforting for a while to buy into the myth that I had no control and that the world was against me, because then I didn't have to confront any of my challenges head-on and make changes.

Living with ADHD can be hard and *debilitating,* and life

can get so overwhelming that you just want to give up entirely, hide under the covers, and settle for the swamp of sadness, but that doesn't have to be your entire story. It doesn't have to say anything about what you're capable of or what you get to do, behave like, or feel in the future. **You can buy into the idea that ADHD means you're doomed to feel like crap forever, or you can buy into the idea that ADHD means that your body and mind operate differently.**

## WHY ARE MANY WOMEN WITH ADHD DIAGNOSED LATER IN LIFE?

According to national data collected by the United States Centers for Disease Control and Prevention (CDC) from 2016 to 2019, boys are almost twice as likely to be diagnosed with ADHD as girls are.

One of the main reasons girls are underdiagnosed is that ADHD often presents differently in females. Rather than being the stereotypical hyperactive kid bouncing around the classroom as many boys are, a lot of girls with ADHD tend to experience their symptoms more internally. While the boy in the classroom was literally running around, it might have been your mind that was doing the racing.

In addition, many women learn how to mask their ADHD and find coping mechanisms to help them manage their symptoms and responsibilities. Sometimes, we might fly under the radar as ambitious high achievers who seem to love a deadline. In reality, though, we might be struggling to stay afloat beneath the surface. As more responsibilities are piled on us in adulthood, there might come a point when our ADHD becomes so unbearable that we realize something is not right and seek answers. We might resort to unhealthy strategies to relieve the internal hyperactivity or look for something to take the pain or stress away. Other diagnoses might start to enter the picture: anxiety, depression, eating disorders, self-harm, addiction. In fact, many women with undiagnosed ADHD are diagnosed with anxiety instead because it's the experience that can be reported on and seen, even though the anxiety is often the result of unmanaged ADHD.

If you suspect you have ADHD, getting a diagnosis will be life-changing. An ADHD diagnosis can bring so much relief because you finally have an answer to why you are the way you are and why you struggle with so many things that other women don't seem to struggle with. Once you realize that there is a reason for your struggles, you can alter your life to work differently.

## WELL-BEING STARTS WITH YOU

When I first started looking at ADHD content on social media, I found plenty of posts telling me what it meant to have ADHD. Many of them were quite negative, gloomy, cynical, and filled with self-deprecating memes and videos. It made me feel disheartened and far from empowered.

Recognizing the troubles we can face as women with ADHD is deeply important, as it helps us understand ourselves better and set up our lives in a way that supports our needs. But believing these troubles have control over us can leave us feeling powerless and weaken our ability to make a change. True well-being can feel so far out of reach when we use most of our energy blaming others for our problems—whether it be the government, modern society, or even family members responsible for pain we experienced in childhood. And, to be clear, we're not *wrong* to be frustrated and hurt by these things. It's just that we have no control over them now. If we truly believe that the only way to be happy is to have something external change—like the passage of new legislation that makes the world cater to those of us with ADHD, or to have that one stubborn person apologize—we can stay stuck and fall into a victim's mentality. We might spend our time waiting for change to happen and blaming outside forces for our problems instead of seizing opportunities to act on what we can change.

Even worse, this defeatist mindset can make it hard for us to take care of ourselves. If we believe we are victims, we will keep finding evidence to confirm this belief. We will spend our lives seeing ourselves as victims of circumstance, wallowing in our pasts and believing we have little power to change anything, thus forever staying the same—unhealthy and unhappy.

But health and happiness don't just happen to us. Because the modern world is so far removed from the world in which our ancestors lived, many of us need to make conscious changes to the way we think and live if we want to do well, feel well, and be well. Believe it or not, well-being is our natural state. But in recent years it's become clear that we are more disconnected from ourselves and the world around us. We've lost the magic of nature, community, connection, and health. We've forgotten how to live in harmony with the world, causing constant stress, and stress is at the root of a lot of physical, mental, emotional, and social diseases. While outside factors affect us, that doesn't mean we should just blame the world and do nothing to change *how we're living in it*.

Taking care of our health and happiness is ultimately a deeply personal and sacred commitment. All we can do is all we can do, and when we feel well, we can positively influence the individuals, groups, society, and world around us for the better if we choose to.

This is why I urge you to opt for an empowered mentality. An empowered mentality helps us see that while we may not have control over the past, we *do* have the ability to shape our own future by making some changes in our current lives.

Instead of waiting for the world to change to suit us, we can decide to create a life that *works for us.* We can take responsibility for what *is* in our control, and feel capable and confident in the process. We see health and happiness as abundant resources, and we choose to move toward them by proactively helping ourselves, regardless of what we've been through in the past. This way of seeing the world is a practice that builds resilience and confidence, so that we can start to move through the world with a sense of purpose, ease, and hope instead of blame and pessimism. When we look at all the (many!) obstacles the world has put in our way, we can say, "Yeah, that all sucks, *and* what can *I* do to feel better?"

---

*Instead of waiting for the world to change to suit us, we can decide to create a life that* works for us.

---

## SEEING YOURSELF AS A WHOLE

As you start thinking about the lifestyle changes that can help you manage ADHD, I encourage you take a 360-degree view of your health and happiness. True wellness requires a biopsychosocial approach. This holistic perspective acknowledges that your thoughts, emotions, and social circumstances play equally crucial roles in shaping your experiences. Here are the factors at play:

- **Biological:** your brain's structure and your body's chemistry and genetics
- **Psychological:** your thoughts, beliefs, and process of making meaning
- **Social:** your home environment, your relationships, and the larger society

Understanding these elements can show you a different approach to well-being, one that gives you the ability to look at your whole self and how you move through the world, opening up more options for addressing your current challenges.

For example, you might find yourself blaming your anxiety on your ADHD (biological). And you would be partially correct! But there are other factors at play. Take a minute to consider your psychological factors—what are your beliefs about your anxiety? Maybe you believe that it's a fixed trait, that you are just "an anxious person." Now, how about your social factors? Maybe your romantic relationship is going through a rough patch and it's leaving you uneasy. Considering every perspective will open new methods of healing. You could try treating the biological factors by exercising or eating more protein to better manage your symptoms. Or maybe you'd prefer to start by rewriting your narrative around anxiety, showing yourself it *is* something that you can heal from. Perhaps you'd rather start your journey by working on your issues with your partner. Suddenly, with this new perspective, you have multiple options at your fingertips. By becoming curious about various aspects of your life, you can better understand your experience and begin to change your narratives about who you are and what is possible for you.

## ONE HABIT AT A TIME

Trying to overhaul many areas of your life can feel overwhelming and lead you to take on too much. When I'm trying to make a change with something as big as my lifestyle, I like to start small with just one habit.

Habits make change more approachable because they allow us to focus on one behavior at a time and make it automatic. They turn something like going for a run from something we actively think about to something we simply do, protecting us from talking our way out of things that are good for us. In fact, neuroscientists have linked habit formation to the basal ganglia, a part of the brain involved in processing emotions, memory, and pattern recognition. Decision-making, on the other hand, happens in a part of the brain called the prefrontal cortex. Once a behavior becomes automatic, the decision-making part of your brain takes a back seat, letting habits run the show.

Building new habits even changes your neural pathways.[*] Thanks to something called neuroplasticity, our brains have the ability to form new neural pathways throughout our lives. Our brains do this automatically when we have a disease or get injured. But we also have the power to intentionally build new pathways by focusing our attention on a new behavior. For example, let's say you used to deal with feelings of stress by overeating, but you recently have decided to try going for a walk instead. The more you repeat the new behavior (walking), the stronger the neural pathways associated with it become. Meanwhile, the neural pathways associated with the old behavior (overeating) will weaken due to decreased use. When neurons stop firing together they lose strength, and the pathway stops activating automatically,

---

[*] Neural pathways are like roads in your brain that help messages move around. They're made of brain cells that talk to one another to control how you think, act, and feel. While having ADHD might mean you face challenges in how information flows along your neural pathways, it's important to remember that these obstacles don't define your ability to form new pathways. Your brain is incredibly adaptable, and it's continuously shaping and adjusting pathways to support your growth and development.

breaking the habit. This is also true when you take a moment before reacting—for example, if you have a habit of responding to a partner's disagreement with immediate defensiveness—pausing before choosing a different response can weaken these old pathways. Over time, you can transform these automatic reactions into more helpful responses and habits. This change happens in the space between the trigger and the response—the pause, the moment before you react.

A single habit change can also serve as a catalyst for even more beneficial changes. **Transformation happens when one habit feeds into another, creating a domino effect.** Say, for instance, that you've decided to make it a habit to finish eating for the day by 8:00 P.M. Thanks to this new habit, you do less late-night eating, which means you feel sleepier earlier in the evening. Going to bed earlier means you wake up feeling more energized the next day. You've always wanted to try running, and now that you feel more refreshed in the morning, you start going for a ten-minute jog after you wake up. To support your new running habit, you begin looking for ways to eat more protein at mealtimes.

Let's be real, though; creating new habits doesn't always feel easy, especially for those of us with ADHD. Because of some developmental differences in our brains, we have trouble with planning, staying organized, and sticking to routines.

## THE DOMINO EFFECT

Finish eating by 8 p.m.

Go to bed earlier

Go for a morning jog

Eat more protein at each meal

Plus, ADHD brains love excitement and novelty, which makes it even harder to create habits.

It takes around sixty-six days to form a new habit.[*] Those first sixty-six days of habit building might feel tough, but habits can be built if we know how they work and how to make them work for our brains. There are creative ways to keep yourself moving forward until the behavioral change you want

---

* One study published in the *European Journal of Social Psychology* in 2009 found it took participants anywhere from 18 to 254 days to form a new habit, with the median time being 66 days. The length of time required to form a habit varied depending on the complexity of the habit and individual differences—such as past experiences, cognitive abilities, and environmental influences. Some naturally had a high level of self-discipline, making it easier for them to stick to a new habit, while others struggled more with self-control and required extra help and more time. Factors such as having a supportive community, stress levels, and your daily routine could also affect how fast you picked up a new habit.

to make becomes more automatic and a part of who you are. I turned to these principles as I explored each pillar covered in this book, and you'll see them in action in each chapter.

## Make a Habit That You Actually Want to Do

Those of us with ADHD have brains that prioritize excitement over importance. We have an interest-driven nervous system wired to focus on what excites us instead of an importance-based nervous system wired to focus on what we actually *need* to do. If you want to establish a habit, the first step is to choose something that actually excites you. Because of this interest-driven nervous system, creating a habit out of necessity isn't enough to motivate us to stick with it. If you force yourself to keep running on the treadmill just because you *should,* even though you hate it, your trips to the gym won't last. Although doing hard things *is* important for brain growth, repeatedly forcing yourself to do things you don't enjoy can leave you feeling resentful and burned out. You're much more likely to keep going if you know yourself and the things that help you enjoy forming new habits.

## ZOOM OUT AND SEE THE BIGGER PICTURE

If you want to understand which habits aren't working for you and get clarity on what you want to do instead, you'll need to take a bird's-eye view of your life. When you're way up in the sky looking down from this perspective, you might notice that you're trying to do multiple things at once—and doing none of them well. You have many passions and responsibilities, and your head is in ten places. Take a moment to answer these questions to help you choose the habit that will make the most impact.

### What You Want to Do

What is one habit that might help you feel more energized, bring better health, or quiet your mind?

_____

_____

Do you want to start practicing this habit? (If no, go back to the previous question and choose a different habit.)

_____

What feeling do you think this habit will bring?

_____

_____

In which part of your day can you most easily engage with this
habit?

_____

_____

## What You Want to Stop Doing

What is one habit that is sapping your energy, hurting your
health, or fogging your mind?

_____

_____

Do you want to keep this habit? (If yes, go back to the previous
question and choose a different habit.)

_____

What feeling does this habit bring?

_____

_____

When do you usually engage with the habit?

_____

_____

Could you replace this old habit with the new one you chose above, *even if it's just for a couple of minutes*?

(If no, move on to the next set of questions.)

_____

## What Is Already Working?

What is one habit you already have and do well that supports your well-being?

_____

_____

Do you want to keep practicing this habit? (If no, go back to the previous question and choose a different habit.)

_____

What feelings does this habit bring?

_____

_____

When do you perform this habit daily?

_____

_____

Can you add performing a new habit to this one to help the new habit stick? (This is called habit stacking; see page 27.) (If no, choose a new habit and repeat.)

_____

_____

## Replace a Habit Instead of *Breaking* a Habit

Breaking old habits takes more effort than starting new ones because once a behavior becomes automatic, it takes a lot of effort to stop engaging in it. This challenge is especially true for those of us with ADHD, because we struggle with impulsivity and self-regulation, making it hard to simply "not" do something. Instead of focusing on stopping a behavior, like *do not eat chocolate when you're stressed,* it's better to select a new behavior to replace it with, like *eat an apple, go for a walk,* or even *eat a handful of nuts with that chocolate.* That's because it's hard to make a habit out of *not doing* something. Instead, replacing an undesirable habit with a new, positive behavior provides a concrete and achievable action. This strategy leverages the natural tendency to take action rather than resisting it, making it easier to build healthier habits.

Think about *adding in* instead of *taking away.* This approach also helps create a sense of accomplishment because when you see yourself making progress with a new behavior, it boosts your confidence and makes you feel more capable of carrying out more healthy changes. Over time, you may begin to link the craving with the new behavior you've incorporated. To borrow from the example we just used, eventually you'll notice that when you feel stressed, you'll crave a walk rather than feel the old desire for chocolate.

## Reframe Routine

Establishing a daily habit on some level requires routine. Now, I know, I know—you *hate* the word "routine." And it's not that you haven't tried! You've spent a lot of time and money on planners and apps, but nothing seems to stick. Every time you try to establish a routine, you feel trapped, stuck, and eventually bored. I get it. I was the queen of telling people I hated doing the same thing every day. That I was too much of a free soul to be tied to something as boring as a routine.

When I look back at some of the healthiest, happiest, and most mentally stable times in my life, there is no denying it. The one commonality they all share is a sense of **routine**. And that's because routine brings clarity and a sense of order. These reduced my feelings of uncertainty and help-lessness, giving me a clearer sense of purpose and direction in my daily life. The funny part is that it's only in looking back on it that I realize I've always had routines in place. I just didn't necessarily consider them routines at the time. I was simply doing things the way I enjoyed doing them. I was happily moving my body every day in ways that felt good and brought me joy. I was drinking a high-protein breakfast shake every day because it was both easy and tasty. I was enjoying eating my Sensory Snack Bowl (see page 160) while winding down at night. These routines didn't match the description of what I thought a "routine" was: rules, boredom, 5:00 A.M. mornings, and a lack of freedom.

I later realized that my definition of "routine" could be different from the one I had subscribed to my whole life. And yours can be too. The words "routine" and "structure" don't need to feel claustrophobic and restrictive. Routines can bring clarity and a sense of order, reducing uncertainty and chaos. You can create a routine and life structure filled with habits you love or transform beneficial habits you *don't* love into ones that you *do* love. (To learn how, read on.)

## Give Yourself Flexibility

Charles Duhigg, author of *The Power of Habit,* explains that every habit has four parts: a cue, an action, a reward, and a craving.

1. **Cue:** The trigger that starts the habit, leading to a craving for the action.

2. **Action:** The action you take in response to the cue, driven by the craving for the reward.

3. **Reward:** The benefit or feeling you get from the action, satisfying the craving that drove the behavior.

4. **Craving:** The intense desire that drives you to repeat the habit and reinforce the pathway in your brain.

I'd like to introduce a fifth element to consider when forming new habits: **flexibility.** Approaching habits with flexibility gives you opportunities to practice the problem-solving and self-compassion you need to *sustain* a long-term lifestyle change. There's no new habit that you will enjoy every single day. You might find some elements of the habit unpleasant. You might not feel motivated a lot of the time. You could question whether you should bother anymore. There will be many parts that you don't enjoy, and that might make you think that the whole healthy-living thing isn't for you. **But guess what? The way you do things can change! In fact, changing the way you practice your habit can keep it fresh and exciting.**

You don't need to do something at the same time, in the same place, and in the same way. To paraphrase Tony Robbins, I want you to stay committed to your vision but be flexible with the approach. If you begin to feel bored by getting the same reward from practicing a habit, change how often you perform the habit and what you reward yourself with. If the thought of the action you take in response to a cue starts to fill you with dread, find ways to make it more enjoyable, or even just bearable, instead of totally giving up on it. To quote entrepreneur Marie Forleo, flexibility makes the obstacles to building habits "figureoutable."

---

*Approaching habits with flexibility gives you opportunities to practice the problem-solving and self-compassion you need to sustain a long-term lifestyle change.*

---

## Stack Your Habit

Habit stacking is a great way to incorporate a new behavior into an existing routine, ideally one that you find easy. It makes it easier to find a place and time to practice the new habit, especially if you're someone who feels like they can't add anything else to their calendar. To start stacking your habits, take a moment to think about what's easy *and* what's hard (or hard to remember).

For example, in the evening in the dark wintertime, I know I usually can't be bothered to cook a high-protein meal; I reach for takeout or junk food instead. Rather than trying to be less tired and more motivated in the evening (which isn't happening), I hack my routine. I find it hard to make a healthy dinner, but I find it *easy* to take my dog for a walk every morning and grab a cup of coffee along the way.

Since I already have a habit of taking my dog for a walk and coffee offers a built-in reward for going on the walk, I attach cooking to this routine. After my coffee, I go across the street to the local butcher and pick up meat for dinner, and since there's no supermarket noise, queues, or stress, I don't mind doing this. When I get home, I don't allow myself to put that meat in the fridge. (This is what I call a dopamine game. We'll learn more about them in the following section.) Instead, I throw it into the slow cooker along with a bunch of herbs and veggies and let it cook at low heat all day. This clears the mental load that comes from thinking about cooking later, and freeing up this brain space feels like a reward in and of itself, becoming something I want to experience again and again. Over time, having a healthy dinner waiting for me became as second nature as picking up a coffee on the way home from walking my dog.

## Play Dopamine Games

Those of us with ADHD are prone to craving instant gratification and gravitate toward activities that give us quick hits of dopamine, a neurotransmitter that helps us feel pleasure and motivation. In most cases, these activities aren't helpful for our well-being: checking social media, eating junk food, provoking arguments with others. They seem like easy, fun options in the moment, but anything that gives you a spike of dopamine without requiring real effort will lead to a subsequent crash in your dopamine levels. This is what often keeps us trapped in a toxic cycle. After a brief high from the activity, your dopamine level drops, leaving you feeling dissatisfied and searching for more dopamine to bring your mood back up again. This is why you find yourself stuck in a social media scroll hole, trying to keep getting that hit. But what are you supposed to do when you feel you have no motivation to cook a healthy meal, but you easily get a tingly feeling of motivation and excitement when you remember you have your favorite ice cream in the freezer?

My solution: Work with your interest-driven nervous system by playing dopamine games to reward yourself with longer-lasting, healthier sensations of pleasure. To play, pick a reward for engaging in your habit but then delay receiving it until you've completed your habit. Let's say you want to start loading the dishwasher before your dishes pile up. At the same time, you have a couple of new Amazon packages stacked near your doorway. The interest-driven part of your brain is going to gravitate toward those packages, seeking the dopamine hit that will come from opening them. Instead of giving in, delay opening the packages until after you've loaded the dishwasher. Suddenly, the mundane task has a fun twist. You can't wait to get through those dishes so you can get that reward of opening the parcels.

Delaying rewards in this way is an incredibly effective tool for establishing a new habit. It helps you prioritize long-term gains over instant gratification. It takes advantage of how the brain's reward system works. Dopamine isn't released only when you receive a reward, but also when you *anticipate* it. This anticipation can lead to an even greater release of dopamine when you receive the reward, turning a task that you don't always feel like doing into something exciting.

You can play dopamine games with almost anything, and there are many different ways to delay rewards. You can infuse little dopamine boosters throughout the process of doing something. Let's say the habit you're trying to establish is running. In reality, all you want to do is go get a coffee and a pastry with a friend. You might choose a running route that ends with meeting your friend at a bakery so you can get your pastry and catch up with your friend immediately after you finish your run. You can even add in little dopamine boosters as you complete your route—getting excited about the reward, varying your route to keep things interesting, or paying attention to how great you feel in the moment while moving.

## NOURISHING YOUR DOPAMINE SYSTEM

A common misconception among ADHD people I talk to or see on social media is that we just have low dopamine levels and producing dopamine is hard for us. But over time, factors such as stress, poor diet, lack of sleep, and a sedentary lifestyle can negatively impact how dopamine works in our brain and the health of our dopamine system. Learning experiences during our formative years can also have an impact. For example, if a frustrated adult repeatedly stepped in to complete a task for you when you were a child and your ADHD was making it difficult for you to focus, that robbed you of the opportunity to experience the reward of having accomplished the task yourself. Repeatedly having encounters like this is just one small way that the brain's sensitivity to dopamine can be affected, including changes in dopamine receptor density or function.

Luckily there are things we can do to nourish the dopamine system we *do* have. When we wake up each morning, our dopamine is at a baseline, and throughout the day, we are constantly replenishing or depleting it, depending on our activities and behavior. If you reach for your phone to scroll through your social media as soon as you wake up, your dopamine levels will have spiked and crashed before you've even gotten out of bed. The possibility of finding something stimulating on your feed keeps you hooked and craving more screen time, leaving you more likely to chase quick and easy dopamine hits from scrolling throughout the rest of the day. That can leave you with a worsened mood, lower motivation, and greater irritability. You can boost your dopamine system function by delaying these types of behavior for as long as possible—for instance, by creating a gap between when you wake up and when you get on social media.

The good news is that you can support the health of your dopamine system. You can positively impact your dopamine function and build a sense of well-being with simple, everyday activities that bring peace, connection, and fulfillment. Think movement, meditation, breathwork, prayer, hiking, watching a sunset, or time with pets, family, and friends who feel good to be around. Even just giving yourself time to chill out can be incredibly effective.

Many people make the mistake of working too hard until they're really tired and then doing something to replenish and relax at the end of the night. Don't let it get to that point. Instead, keep your cup full by consciously choosing to engage in these healthy dopamine-boosting activities before your reserve hits zero. They can be a powerful way to enhance your ability to experience satisfaction, making little, everyday activities more enjoyable and contributing to both a positive outlook and a greater sense of fulfillment in life.

## Keep Your Eyes on the Prize

We are not forming new habits to reach a specific goal and then call it a day. We are forming them so we can begin falling in love with our lives. Short-term goals, such as shedding five pounds or running a marathon, are all milestones to celebrate, but if we mistake them for the destination, we will simply stop practicing the habits that got us there and wind up back at square one, aimless, unhealthy, and unhappy.

So then, what *is* the end goal? It's to continually challenge yourself to see what's possible, to see how good you can feel, and to find out how good life can get. More important, it's to *believe* that you can fall in love with your life. Every single thing in your life doesn't have to change in order for you to fall in love with it. Your life right now, exactly as it is, ADHD and all, has the potential to be this wonderful.

**You can have ADHD *and* be healthy and happy.** In fact, the way our brains operate comes with many strengths that will help us in creating our best lives. We are often very creative, which means we can come up with new ways to form our habits and find work-arounds for challenges. When life inevitably throws obstacles our way, we're good at adapting to changes, allowing us to adjust our habits as needed. And even though we sometimes have trouble keeping our attention on one thing, the hyperfocus we have on the things that interest us can help us build a life we love. Impulsivity is a form of efficiency—when handled right. As people with ADHD, we are usually very enthusiastic about the things we like. We can use this excitement to keep us motivated throughout the process.

ADHD doesn't have to be a limitation. Sure, you can decide, *I have ADHD. That's why my life sucks.* But you can also choose to think, *I have ADHD, and I'm going to use it to my advantage as I create the very best life for myself, one full of health and happiness.*

> **Q:** I have ADHD. My basal ganglia and prefrontal cortex obviously aren't working right because I find it impossible to make good decisions and form new habits. Are the changes that you're sharing in this chapter even possible for me?
>
> **A:** I know it might not seem like it when you're feeling down, but you really *can* optimize your health and help your brain run more efficiently. Many of the lifestyle shifts presented in this book will help with this: regularly exercising, eating a balanced diet, getting good-quality sleep, effectively managing stress, challenging your brain, nurturing social connections, avoiding alcohol and drug use, practicing mindfulness, and trying brain-healthy supplements after consulting with a professional. I know that might feel like an overwhelming list, but each of these practices—alongside the others we will

discuss throughout this book—is a new opportunity to improve your health.

If you're still not convinced, I'd like to tell you about the law of accumulation, one of the greatest success principles of all time. This law says that everything in life is an accumulation of thousands of tiny efforts that nobody ever sees. Not only does every successful attempt to practice a good habit count, but all the little moments that didn't go your way also make a difference. All you need to do is try, and to try something different if it doesn't work out the first time. When you're putting together a puzzle, you might not know where to start, so you just put two pieces together. They may not fit, but you keep trying with other pieces with the belief that you'll eventually figure out how they all fit together.

So, start at your own pace, picking the practices that feel appealing to you in the moment. Slowly but surely, you'll notice the healthy habits building and how you feel about yourself improving.

# 2

## Practice Self-Compassion

*You can hold yourself accountable without
treating yourself like an asshole.*

Think of a woman with ADHD whom you deeply admire.
This can be someone you're close to in real life or someone you enjoy following online. Imagine that this woman
has arrived late to her yoga class and her teacher doesn't let
her into the class. She feels frustrated and annoyed with herself, but this isn't the first thing that has gone wrong this
week. She forgot to do meal prep last night. She made a mistake on a work project, and her co-worker is being difficult
about it. The stress from the last few days has been building
up, and exercise is the one thing that truly regulates her
mood. This was the only time this week that she had for a
class, and as she stands in the lobby of the studio, she's on
the brink of a meltdown.

You call her up and tell her: *You should have known better.
You screw this up all the time, and you need to get your shit together and stop being lazy. It's so embarrassing. There are plenty*

*of people who have way more responsibility than you, and you can't even make it to a class on time.*

She says nothing in response. You hang up the phone.

Imagine the look on her face and her body language as the words you spewed repeat in her mind. Pay attention to how she is unable to shake them off.

What do you think she will do next? Will she decide to try again, book another class, and then get on with her day? Or will she go home, eat ice cream to cope, and make herself feel even worse because she thinks you're right? Will she say to herself, *What's the point? I am lazy, and there's no point in trying. This is just another failure of a day.*

I know you wouldn't say hateful things like this to other women with ADHD.

So why do you say those things to yourself?

If you don't admire yourself the way you admire others, it's time to change that. Cultivating self-compassion and moving away from critical self-talk will form the foundation of everything we do in *Healthy Happy ADHD*.

## THERE'S A DIFFERENCE BETWEEN PRACTICING ACCOUNTABILITY AND BULLYING YOURSELF

Self-compassion is the first pillar of *Healthy Happy ADHD* because without it, you'll never give yourself a chance. In times of change, you need encouragement and kindness, especially from yourself. Those of us with ADHD can be really hard on ourselves; we can be overly self-critical and expect a level of perfection we wouldn't impose upon others. We often suffer from low self-esteem and have high expectations for how much we think we *should* be able to do from day to day and how easy it *should* feel. We are often our own worst critics, and living in a world not always set up to be ADHD-friendly gives us so many reasons to be hard on ourselves.

*In times of change, you need encouragement and kindness, especially from yourself.*

The reality is, you're not going to get everything perfect every single time, every single day. There will be times when you feel totally defeated or that you've messed up. You will forget habits, and you will fall off track. In moments like these, **it's often the self-critical voice in your head that makes it easy to give up on yourself, which isn't fair to your goals and dreams**. That negative self-talk can lead to self-sabotage, deepening the *What's the point?* mentality that keeps you looking for quick fixes instead of long-term shifts.

Self-compassion gives you another path. It allows you to hold yourself accountable *without* the self-bullying that so often leads to giving up entirely. **By being kind to yourself when you've failed or didn't perform as well as you wanted to, you will be able to weather the ups and downs when you have a bad day or things don't go as planned.** It offers you the chance to learn from those tough moments and to use that wisdom to help yourself move forward so that when they happen again, you'll be better prepared. Rather than beating yourself up while ignoring the hurt you feel, you can acknowledge your feelings and notice the words you're speaking to yourself. In that process, you give yourself support, space, and love. You deepen the relationship that you hold with yourself.

## BELIEVE IT OR NOT, YOU'RE WORTHY OF COMPASSION

A lot of the criticisms you have of yourself are the result of old patterns in your brain and nervous system that you haven't broken yet. You don't sit there and decide, *Okay, now I am going to think about how crap I am.* It's more likely that the thought just seamlessly pops into your head.

This thought doesn't need to mean anything about you as a person, though. It's just something floating around in your head, trying to become relevant. Thoughts hold only as much meaning as you give them. As Daniel Amen, MD, says, "Don't believe every stupid thing you think."

Sometimes our "bad" habits—the distraction, the avoidance, the procrastination that we experience in our everyday lives—are coping mechanisms that we developed long ago because they kept us safe as children. Your brain created a coping mechanism to keep you safe and help you handle overwhelming emotions in moments when you felt threatened or unsafe. Maybe your schoolwork was harshly criticized as a child, so you avoid the pain of potential failure by procrastinating on tasks that need to be done. Maybe you witnessed something traumatic at a young age, causing you to dissociate or disconnect from reality as a way to cope with overwhelming fear. Maybe you were raised in an environment where emotions were disregarded or dismissed, leading you to suppress or deny your own feelings and basic needs to avoid appearing vulnerable.

Whatever it was, you might carry that same coping mechanism with you into adulthood, even though it's no longer serving you the way it once did. Now, instead of keeping you safe, this coping mechanism interferes with your day-to-day life.

Think of your brain as a computer system. The negative behavior you're so harsh with yourself about isn't a character flaw; it's just a result of some outdated programming—programming that was coded when you were a child, possibly even passed down to you by generations before you. The system is simply outdated at this point in your life. It's time for an update.

## How to Talk to Yourself

Your brain has a built-in GPS that helps you find the best route to your destination, whatever it may be. It's always moving toward your goals, even if you think you don't have any. Best of all, this internal GPS is equipped to learn from mistakes. When you let this natural learning process take place, it will start directing you to approaches, tools, and opportunities that work better for you.

When you have a bad day, when the work doesn't go as planned, or when you feel like you've messed up, negative self-talk can send your thoughts spiraling, interrupting this natural learning process. While you can't get rid of negative thoughts altogether, you can prevent this spiral from distracting your brain from its GPS by shifting the narrative that you create from these thoughts. You have a great imagination, so when it's taking off in the wrong direction, do a U-turn and get back on the road toward becoming your best self by practicing these five steps:

1. The next time you catch yourself saying something nasty to yourself, **notice** your thoughts and bring them

to your conscious awareness. In that moment, the thoughts might feel rough, emotional, and even irrational, especially if they have compounded over time. Notice whether any physical sensations accompany these thoughts; areas of tension or discomfort in your body may be manifestations of emotional distress.

2. **Accept** what happened for what it is. Our minds often want to dwell on even the simplest mistake, like arriving a few minutes late to a yoga class. And, while we don't want to minimize our experiences, we also don't want to build them into more than what they are. Rather than taking every negative thing you think about yourself seriously or forcing yourself to think positively about the situation, try simply acknowledging what happened. (*It happened. What's done is done, and how I feel is how I feel.*)

3. **Feel compassion** toward yourself because you know you're doing your best. When you find yourself being particularly self-critical, remember that example we discussed at the beginning of the chapter. Think back to the woman with ADHD whom you admire, who's working hard at bettering herself. If she had a bad week, would you be harsh and tell her that she's awful, that she's never going to achieve her goals? I highly

doubt that. More likely, you would remind her that she's doing her best. That one setback or mistake does not define her. If she is worthy of this reassurance, you are worthy too. **You deserve the same grace you give your loved ones.** (*ADHD makes things hard. I am learning, I am doing my best in each moment, and as I move through new changes, my confidence is growing every day.*)

4. **Forgive** yourself as quickly as you can instead of directing unnecessary anger at yourself. I know how hard you are on yourself, and it's killing your spirit. You deserve better. The beautiful thing about self-compassion is that it opens the door for self-forgiveness. Once we can forgive ourselves for our mistakes, we dial down the self-punishment for every little slipup and cut ourselves some slack. We can realize that our mistakes were just that—mistakes. And from there we can move on. (*I forgive myself for having blind spots. I learn from them; they don't make me a bad person. I let go of my anger at myself. I trust that I am making great progress, even when I fall off track.*)

5. **Move forward** and know that the vision you have for your healthier lifestyle and where you want to be *is still going to happen*. Will your path be perfect? Quick?

Easy? Like everyone else's? No, no, and no. But is your success absolutely, inevitably going to happen without a shred of a doubt? Yes. **Instead of living in the past, you are now heading toward the future.** (*I move forward. I am still committed to my vision and know that success is still on the horizon. I have the power to shape what happens next, and I'm ready to move forward and do the next best thing.*)

## THE FIVE STEPS TO SELF-COMPASSION

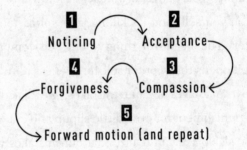

It's going to take some time to change the way you speak to yourself. The moments when you need positive self-talk and self-compassion the most will also be the times when they're hardest to practice. This is all absolutely okay. It will take your brain a while to catch up with these ideas as you condition yourself to feel different, forgive, and move forward with hope after a setback.

Take this recent experience I had as an example. I woke up

late on the morning of an apartment viewing after staying up too late the night before. I was tired, my mood was low, and I ended up being late for my 10:00 A.M. appointment with a real estate agent. I had emailed to say I'd be ten minutes late, then emailed again at 9:50 to say I'd be on time, only to show up at 10:11 because I took a wrong turn. The agent was annoyed with me, but I was even more annoyed with myself. My self-talk turned nasty: *I'm a mess. Why couldn't I just leave on time? I shouldn't have made that wrong turn. Why do I have to make everything harder than it needs to be? He thinks I'm an idiot. This is embarrassing.*

The bad feelings lingered for the rest of the day and completely turned it upside down. It wasn't until later that day when I was sitting on the sofa that I realized I was holding on to a lot of unnecessary anger at myself, and at this stranger, the realtor, guessing what he might or might not think of me. The first step that I took to process this angry feeling was to notice my thoughts. To keep moving out of this anger, I ran through the next four steps—acceptance, self-compassion, forgiveness, and forward motion. *It is what it is. I have ADHD. I am under a lot of pressure right now, and the overwhelm was clouding my ability to think straight or be on time for anything. I have been finding life hard lately, but I am still doing my best.* Rather than clinging to a moment I can't change, I can allow myself to feel the way I feel and then redirect my energy toward making a positive change in my life.

## REFRAMING NEGATIVE SELF-TALK

*This is so embarrassing. I'm late again, and they think I'm an idiot.*
→ I am late because I have ADHD. I'd like to get better with punctuality, but some days I find it hard. I am doing my best. I am doing my best. I am doing my best.

*Everyone is so much further ahead.* → I am exactly where I need to be. Everything is always working out for me, and I must remember that I have ADHD. I am exactly where I need to be and trust I am moving in the right direction.

*This is the tenth time I've made this mistake.* → It's taking me longer than expected to get the hang of this, but I'm getting there faster than before.

*If I had just stuck to that one thing, I'd be more successful by now.* → My curious ADHD mind loves trying new things. My curiosity is an asset. As the saying goes, "A jack of all trades is a master of none, but oftentimes better than a master of one."

## How to Stay Accountable with Questions, Not Criticism

As you practice the five steps to self-compassion, you might notice that there are patterns, behaviors, and habits that you'd like to understand more deeply. For example, maybe you miss every single workout class you book and end up in a spiral of negative feelings about yourself. While you now know how to stop yourself from plummeting further into the spiral, you're not sure how to get to the root of your behavior without your inner critic spewing venom. Your mind might be accustomed to telling you that you missed your class because you are "lazy," "unfit," or "careless."

As much as your mind might try to convince you otherwise, it's often the case that the mistakes you made are not actually the most important piece of the puzzle. What *really* matters is the interpretation you attach to those mistakes and how those interpretations affect the way you see yourself. When you view each slipup as a confirmation of your shortcomings, that viewpoint reinforces negative beliefs about yourself and slows the creation of positive neural pathways in your brain. If you want to stop believing you're lazy, unfit, or careless, the first step is to stop calling yourself "lazy," "unfit," or "careless." No matter how many workout classes you miss.

Rather than tuning in to self-criticism, I invite you to have a conversation with yourself. Your goal is to analyze your behavior without attaching any judgments, criticisms, or feelings about what this behavior means about you.

Ask yourself these questions, and answer them honestly. Don't be afraid of what you find.

- Why do I feel bad about what happened? *I feel bad for missing the workout class because I want to get fit.*

- How often does this happen? *This happens multiple times a week.*

- What seems to be getting in the way? *I'm exhausted in the evenings.*

- Can I do something else right now to replace what I missed? *I could go for a long walk.*

- How can I make what I want to do easier next time? *Instead of booking a class for right after work, when I am tired from working with people all day, I could try a morning class, before work.*

Asking yourself questions in a nonjudgmental way might feel difficult at first, especially when your brain has grown so accustomed to reflexively berating yourself every time you make a mistake. But you need to make the shift if you truly want to progress. The right questions have the potential to change your life, and you'll be surprised by the ideas and solutions you come up with. Each time you have these little conversations with yourself, you'll explore why you do what you do. This information is valuable, and you'll use it to tweak your routines to make them work for you instead of forcing yourself to adopt a way of being and functioning that doesn't suit you. You'll start to think more clearly, and slowly but surely, shift the way you see yourself, and the results you get.

# FINDING SOLUTIONS FOR SETBACKS

**The setback: I ate fast food for dinner.**

- Why do I feel bad about what happened? *I feel bad about eating fast food for dinner. I want to eat healthier and take care of my body.*

- How often does this happen? *This happens three or four times a week.*

- What seems to be getting in the way? *I don't eat all day because of stress in the office, so I'm starving by the time I finish work and don't have the capacity to cook.*

- Can I do something else right now to replace what I missed? *I can go for a walk now to help my digestion and energy level.*

- How can I make what I want to do easier next time? *I can keep some protein powder, nut butter, and seeded crackers at my desk for convenience to ensure I'm eating food during busy days, which will help me stop bingeing on fast food in the evening.*

**The setback: I arrived late to work.**

- Why do I feel bad about what happened? *I feel annoyed because I'm working toward a promotion and I don't want my boss to think I don't care.*

- How often does this happen? *This happens most Mondays and Fridays.*

- What seems to be getting in the way? *Traffic en route to my office is always heavy in the mornings.*

- Can I do something else right now to replace what I missed? *No, I can't undo the fact that I was late, but I can set aside time at lunch to think about what I can do to make it easier to arrive on time.*

- How can I make what I want to do easier next time? *To make it easier for myself, I could try another commuting option, such as carpooling, taking public transit, or cycling to work, so I don't need to worry about traffic.*

**The setback: I missed yoga class.**

- Why do I feel bad about what happened? *I feel annoyed about missing yoga because I prepaid for my spot.*

- How often does this happen? *This happens most of the time when I am frazzled and stressed.*

- What seems to be getting in the way? *This studio doesn't allow latecomers. The door is always locked at 5:59 P.M. on the dot.*

- Can I do something else right now to replace what I missed? *I could stream a fifteen-minute class online. There are a few instructors I enjoy following.*

- How can I make what I want to do easier next time? *To make it easier, I could avoid booking at this studio because I know that I am often a couple of minutes late.*

## YOU DEFINE YOUR PATH

Practicing self-compassion is more than just changing the way we talk to ourselves. We also need to change how we think about the path ahead of us and view it through a more flexible lens. Many of us with ADHD have rigid ideas about what change looks like or believe there is a "right" way to make it happen. We have a habit of taking other people's opinions as markers for how we *should* think and the goals we should and shouldn't have for ourselves.

The problem with sticking to these ideas is that we then stop thinking for ourselves. We override our own values, ignore our inner guidance and intuition, and hide what we want. We might ignore what is important to us and what excites us in order to fit in.

In reality, there's no scorecard to fill out, no exam to pass or fail, and no one to answer to—except yourself. You have the freedom to do things in a way that works for you and your brain and your daily life. But knowing that you have this freedom might not be enough to stop you from doubting yourself or feeling as if your approach to your journey is wrong. When I went through my transformation, here are the insights that helped me the most when I treated myself harshly for what I was doing and where I was headed.

## See Yourself as Someone to Love Instead of Someone to Fix

One of the reasons it can be hard to make peace with the path we need to take is internalized shame. Shame is an important emotion. It helps us evaluate our own behavior, gain a clear understanding of what's wrong and what's right, and figure out how to live in harmony with society, but when we begin feeling shame for things about ourselves that aren't inherently wrong or bad, it can warp our self-image, making us feel inadequate and convincing us that we are not worthy of kindness.

For many of us with ADHD, shame about our way of being begins in childhood. When we were little, we might have been told or shown that being yourself is just not a good idea. Our ADHD-related struggles might have caused us to make mistakes or fail to meet the expectations of parents, teachers, friends, and the world at large. When shame goes unaddressed for a long period of time, it becomes internalized. You can start to believe that you are deeply flawed, worthless, inadequate, and unlovable. This sense of internalized shame often comes up when we use the word "should," as in *I'm not as smart as I should be. I'm not as organized as I should be. I should have my shit together at this point. I should be able to handle this. I shouldn't have dressed like that. I shouldn't leave all this dirty laundry out if people are coming over.* We push ourselves to make positive changes in our lives as a result of fear, self-criticism, or a sense of unworthiness.

You can make changes to your external world and your busy schedule, move more, and eat well, but you won't resolve the core problems that affect your quality of life unless you stop seeing yourself as the enemy. You are not flawed or broken. Your body and brain are not letting you down or attacking you. Everything they have been doing has arisen from a desire to protect you and help you survive your current circumstances. **Badgering yourself about all the ways in which you're not good enough or treating yourself like a problem to solve only keeps your body in a heightened state of stress. You'll be more successful at breaking free of the vicious cycle if you're doing it because you love and care for yourself rather than because you believe you need to fix yourself.**

Thankfully, there is a better way. One of the simplest ways we can treat ourselves with kindness, understanding, and acceptance is to replace the "should" statements with acknowledgments of our struggles and mistakes, allowing us to focus on practicality and self-care rather than self-judgment. Improve your health because you genuinely want to take care of yourself, manage your ADHD symptoms, and feel better, not because of a sense of shame or self-hatred.

## REFRAMING THE "SHOULDS"

*I should pick up this dirty laundry if people are coming over.* → It's okay if there's some dirty laundry out when people come over; it would be helpful to put it away, but I don't have the energy to tackle it right now.

*I should have my shit together at this point.* → I'm learning and growing at my own pace, and it's okay if I don't have everything figured out at this age.

*I should have dressed differently had I known who was coming.* → My outfit choice felt good to me, and it was a reflection of my personal style, mood, and sense of comfort at that moment. That's perfectly valid.

## It's Okay to Want to Change

Seeing yourself as someone to love doesn't necessarily mean that the way you live your life is perfect as is. If you don't like how you feel, think, and behave right now, the idea of making changes might feel right, even exciting. Wanting to change doesn't mean that you don't respect who you are. In fact, the opposite is true.

I came to this realization after I woke up feeling bloated after a few too many nights of late-night takeout. Getting dressed for my reformer Pilates class was a struggle. Everything felt tight in all the wrong places, worsening my sensory issues. My mood was low. I felt annoyed with myself for not taking care of myself and tired because the food I had been choosing to eat was upsetting my tummy. I stumbled slowly down the stairs and caught a glimpse of my swollen face in the mirror. I felt sick and lethargic, as if nothing in my body was working right.

Instead of berating myself for all the unhealthy nights of takeout or telling myself, *This is who I am now, and this is who I will always be,* I chose to be kind to myself. Being kind to myself didn't mean I got back into my bed, ordered more food, and stopped exercising forever. It meant acknowledging that I never wanted to feel this way again. In that moment, I decided it was time for a change. This time, I meant it.

My career as a health and fitness coach has taught me that it's not only possible to change, it's that the pursuit of change can help us feel a deeper level of love and respect for ourselves than ever before. Moments like the one I described can show you what you no longer want to tolerate from yourself and how you can begin to see change as an act of love. The reality is that many of us want to experience the vibrancy of life, and we simply can't do that if we treat ourselves like trash. If you're struggling and overwhelmed, you can change without believing that something is wrong with you. Trust me, you are capable. You will feel that joyful vibrancy soon.

## Find Peace in the Imperfect Process

A lot of your work with self-compassion will ask you to embrace this fact: You have ADHD. While there are ways to reduce its negative impact so you can live in harmony with yourself and the world around you, you won't necessarily *remove* it from your life. Because you have ADHD, the process of becoming healthier and happier won't always be smooth sailing. As someone with ADHD and as a coach, I can say from firsthand experience that there are a lot of speed bumps, but I like to remind myself and my clients that **speed bumps aren't roadblocks.** They may slow you down, but they do not have the power to stop you or bring you to a dead end.

Sometimes life as an ADHD woman means you miss a workout or you have dessert for dinner. Ultimately, in the grand scheme of things, it doesn't matter, so put your energy somewhere other than berating yourself for "messing up." Get on with it, find new perspectives, try new ways of doing things, and keep moving forward with your goals, because that's who you are and that's what you do.

Understanding that ADHD makes many things harder and will make it take longer for you to achieve your desired results is a key part of moving forward. In fact, how quickly you can get over a setback and bounce back from defeat is what will determine the speed of your transformation, not concentrating on the pursuit of perfection. In fact, avoiding mistakes in pursuit of perfection might actually slow your progress because it doesn't leave room for your internal GPS to learn.

You are human and you will struggle, and from that you will grow. There is no shame in that. Right now, you might feel discomfort about being a new runner on the road, but this discomfort helps you become the version of yourself that you want to bring to life. It's temporary. Eventually that version of yourself won't feel the discomfort anymore. You'll have so many moments when you fall down, feel like crap, and then move forward, but know that it is normal to have these feelings when you're trying to establish new habits.

## WHAT DO YOU WANT TO TELL YOUR YOUNGER SELF?

Life can be hard, and we can get so caught up in our stress that we don't recognize that we already have so much that we once wished for. While your life might not be perfect and you might not feel like you have everything together, your younger self would be beaming with excitement if she saw the life you get to live today. We can get so flustered about the future that we sometimes forget about the magic in our lives. This timeline visualization exercise can help you connect with this magic. To be clear, you're not being asked to reconnect with painful memories from your past in this exercise. You're simply sharing the fun parts of your life with that younger version of yourself who would feel awe at things you often take for granted.

Relax and close your eyes. Go back in time and meet your ten-year-old self. Sit with her. Tell her who you are. Tell her all the good things about your life. For example, share that you get to ride your bike to work and go to the cinema *whenever you want*. That purple is still your favorite color. That you still love painting and you do it every day.

Watch her happy face as you tell her about fun parts of your life. Try to stick with the parts of your life that you know will excite her, the parts that might feel magical to a child. You can leave out the work drama—after all, your younger self is only ten.

Watch her face light up with excitement because she thinks you're so cool. She wants you to be her big sister.

Tell her that she gets to *be* you when she's older. As she freaks out with excitement, smile, knowing that you are exactly where you're meant to be, living out the life that the little you dreamed of in so many little ways.

Tell her that you see her, you understand her, and you love her. And that you will not bully her when she grows up. You will be kind to her. You will practice patience. You will love her because you know that's exactly what that little girl deserves and wants from you—and, at the end of the day, it's also what you deserve. You are her, and she is you.

**Q:** When I open social media or hear about someone else's success, I get so stressed out. I start being so hard on myself about my lack of progress. How do I deal with constant comparison?

**A:** The comparison trap is sneaky, and it can come out of nowhere. While I was making one of my favorite pre-gym snacks—butter, almond butter, banana, and honey on toast— I opened Instagram to check the class schedule for my gym and found myself reading a caption from a fellow debut author who recently launched her book.

One caption wasn't enough, so I went to her account and binged on a half-dozen posts. Her beautiful outfits, her consistent daily posting, all the comments, the excitement, the nonstop chatter about the book—I was so engrossed that I forgot about my snack. It was only when a noise in the hallway caught my attention that I snapped out of my trance and remembered what I was supposed to be doing: making toast.

I felt sick with anxiety after just a few minutes of scrolling. I'd been dealing with the imposter syndrome that comes with being a first-time author, and this Instagram post was the perfect cue for the negative self-talk to start: *I'm not posting enough on Instagram. I need to build a community faster. I need to post cute pics. Taking a break from Instagram to focus on writing was a stupid idea. I AM DOING IT ALL WRONG.*

I knew that if I fell into the comparison trap, self-compassion would be my escape route. As I buttered my cold toast, I quickly worked on reframing my thoughts: *Yes, you're anxious. It's normal to feel scared as a first-timer in a new space. I know this is your dream and you don't want to mess it up, but you're not messing it up. You're right on time, doing it your way. You've done some great writing today, and that is what is important. God doesn't call the qualified, he qualifies the called. You're feeling these feelings so you can help others overcome the same roadblocks. You're okay, you're safe. Now eat your toast and go to the gym to move your way through some of this anxious energy.*

Your way doesn't need to look like everyone else's. You aren't obligated to cook like someone without ADHD, to have energy like they do, to have your life together like they do. You don't need to mindlessly scroll while waiting for toast or waiting for anything. The toast tastes better hot. Don't let it go cold because you were looking through someone else's window, trying to see how they cook theirs.

# 3

■

# Change How You See Yourself

*We see ourselves as who we were*
*instead of who we could be.*

Have you ever decided you wanted something and then all of a sudden it seems to be everywhere? Say it's a yellow jacket and you want to buy one for yourself. You might notice someone wearing one or one on display in a store window as you run errands. The fashion influencer you follow might post a photo of herself wearing one, or maybe your co-worker walks into the office with the jacket. It's not that there are suddenly more yellow jackets around. It's that your brain brings yellow jackets to your attention. It puts blinders on for other colors of jackets because you've made a mental note that yellow jackets are important to you.

Your brain will do the same with your beliefs about yourself. It will support those beliefs, whether they're negative or positive, and how you see yourself drives your behavior. If you want your new habits to last and bring the results you are dreaming about, you need to start by changing your beliefs about who you are.

## UNPACKING THE BELIEFS THAT KEEP YOU STUCK

**The key to long-term change—change that sticks—starts with identity work, the process of changing your self-identity and the way you see yourself.** The practice of seeing yourself achieving your goals, overcoming any and all obstacles along the way and getting new results, is all part of identity work.

You will always act in alignment with how you see yourself and who you believe you are. If you believe you're a lucky person, you're more likely to notice all the synchronicities in your life and to act on the opportunities they bring you, the way you expect a lucky person would act. On the other hand, if you believe that you're unlucky, you're more likely to notice when things go wrong and to avoid opportunities that seem risky. Similarly, if you have a victim mentality and believe you're incapable of change, your brain will constantly look for things around you to support that belief.

All of this often happens unconsciously. If left to its own devices, your brain will think the same thoughts and follow the same patterns of behavior every day. This autopilot mode is your brain's way of making life easier for you. It's how it performs its number one job: keeping you safe by flagging potential threats.

**One way that your brain will protect you is by resisting change, even if that means choosing a familiar hell over an unfamiliar heaven.** The reason for this dates all the way back to our evolutionary history. Change represents uncertainty and, although society has evolved past the time when many of us had to worry that a lion might attack us if we took a new route back to our hut at night, our brain is still hardwired to perceive any sort of uncertainty as a threat. This activates our body's stress responses. We'll go over what these stress responses are in chapter 8, but they are the reason that we sometimes feel our heart rate pick up speed and our chest tighten at even just the thought of change.

Rather than embracing change, our brain instead prefers familiar routines and automatic habits because they're easier, more predictable, and less risky. As we touched upon in the last chapter, a lot of these habits were developed when we were very young. If we experienced distress as children, our brains adapted to protect us from experiencing the same distress in the future. Sometimes the roots of these habits can go back even further than our childhood, stemming from generational trauma passed down by family members.

Our brain will often "protect" us from change by bringing up past experiences related to the change that we're trying to make. For instance, if you're considering taking up a new group sport, your brain might remind you of a past experience when you felt embarrassed or inadequate in a team setting. As you recall this past experience and how it felt, thoughts that match the emotional state you are in will bubble up as well. You might notice that when you're sad, you're prone to experiencing more sad thoughts. When you're angry, you're prone to experiencing more angry thoughts. These thoughts then influence your behavior and actions, which leads to outcomes that create more of the same thoughts, and so on. This revolving door of self-reinforcing thoughts and actions keeps going around and around, helping your mind do what it does best: create future situations *based on the past*. **We see ourselves as who we were instead of *who we could be*.** And if we see ourselves as who we were instead of who we *could* be, we find it hard to change. We might struggle to believe that change is possible for us. When we mindlessly use the bad times of the past to predict what will happen in the future, we feel anxious. We might feel that it's not safe to have what we desire or to believe that we can be different and feel different. When we don't feel this sense of possibility or safety, we will simply keep repeating the same actions and getting the same results.

If you see yourself as someone who never gets results, your belief will drive you to behave in ways that lead to the outcome you expect, creating a self-fulfilling prophecy. You might find yourself admitting, *I knew nothing would change. It never does.* As it was put simply by Henry Ford, "Whether you think you can or can't, you're right."

Internalized shame can make matters even worse. As we discussed in the last chapter, those of us with ADHD might carry shame about how we live in and move through the world. We're not only more likely to feel inadequate and begin seeking reasons to support our sense that we are weird or don't belong, we're also more likely to avoid trying the hard, uncomfortable things that will help us change our lives for the better. We might be afraid of putting ourselves in situations where we might make mistakes and fail to meet other people's expectations. We might feel deep down that if people see our true selves and how often we struggle, they will be disappointed in or even disgusted by us.

**The good news is that our belief systems aren't fixed.** The brain makes pathways based on what we think and do the most. The way you feel today and the life you're living today result from your past emotions, thoughts, and actions. The life you'll live tomorrow will also be a result of past emotions, thoughts, and actions. So try something new. The key to making a change is to go from mindlessly *being* to *observing*. You can observe your inner world and see what needs to change so you can build your best future, just as you might record and watch a video of yourself working out at the gym to see how you can improve your form. You can take inventory of your past and decide what thoughts need to change to build your best future.

---

*The key to making a change is to go from mindlessly being to observing.*

---

Are you unhappy in your life? Rather than pushing the answer to that question away, let it rise to the surface. Examine your answer. If you're unhappy, *what* are you unhappy with? Maybe you've lost your love for life and complain endlessly. Maybe you're sick of feeling sluggish in the mornings. Maybe you're over feeling stuck and wallowing in self-pity. Once you give yourself permission to acknowledge what's at the root of your unhappiness, you have the opportunity to start dreaming up a better reality. What kind of person do you *want* to be, how do you *want* to feel, and what do you *want* your days to look like? As you envision this new reality, notice the stories and reactions that surface. When you can, remind yourself that you are choosing to replace old thought patterns with new ones. **Keeping your focus on the better days ahead isn't something that comes easily to you—and it doesn't need to. It's a practice, and over time that practice will become simply part of who you are.**

## CHANGE BEGINS WITH CHOOSING
## YOUR FUTURE SELF

For a lot of people, if a task is important to them and they feel that it *should* be done, they'll likely do it, especially if there's a consequence if they don't.

As someone with ADHD, you have an interest-driven nervous system. You're more likely to do well on a task and to stay motivated when there's deep interest, novelty, and emotion involved. **Knowing that healthy habits are important for managing your ADHD won't be enough for you to make them last. What you need instead is a feeling of excitement and pleasure that you can easily tap into.**

One of the most powerful ways to tap into these feelings is by visualizing your future self. Creating a vision of your future self—who she is, where she is, what she is doing, and how she *feels*—and connecting with how being your future self *feels* can give you a powerful source of motivation that works for the ADHD brain.

Envisioning our future selves is an exercise we can repeat without getting bored because of the many possibilities we can explore. If you wind up forgetting them anyway, there are ways to remember them again. (We'll discuss ideas later in this chapter in "Remember Her," page 88.) More important, having this vision makes the process of change rewarding and satisfying. You will no longer be following habits just because they are important. You will be following them because they help you become the future self you've imagined and it *feels good* to move toward that future. Because it feels good (giving you a boost of dopamine), it becomes easier to choose your future self over your past self. And transformation happens when you keep choosing your future self over your past self.

---

*Transformation happens when you keep choosing your future self over your past self.*

---

When I started practicing regular movement every day to manage my ADHD, I pictured a future where I was fit, healthy, and happy. I had a trip to Miami on my calendar, and I used it to create an image of my future self. I saw her walking along that beach in Miami, smiling, grabbing a coffee before her twenty-minute workout. I saw and *felt* details like the sand on my feet, the first sip of coffee in the sun, and, more important, the *feeling* of confidence and radiance. Doing this also brought me a sense of novelty. This novelty gave me the motivation to start practicing more regular movement, and remembering her kept me going on days when I fell off track and needed motivation to bounce back.

By choosing your future self, you begin showing yourself that it's possible to see yourself in a new light, make changes, undergo transformation, and feel more peace and calm in your life. When you're clear about the identity you want to embody, it's easier to align your behaviors and habits. I've felt trapped and powerless too many times to mention, but I now know I can get out of a rut by consciously deciding that I want better for my future self. I'm still learning, I'm still breaking old patterns, and I still struggle with things, but **when I choose to challenge my beliefs about what's possible, I get to move forward and find the magic that is always waiting for me on the other side.**

## THE BRAIN-ACTIVATING EFFECTS OF VISUALIZATION

Visualization—closing our eyes and really envisioning who we want to be and how we want to feel—is one of the most powerful tools we have at our disposal. This is because of how it works with different parts of the brain.

Visualization not only triggers the reticular activating system (RAS) in your brain, it also activates various brain regions associated with sensory processing, motor planning, and emotional responses. Your RAS is a web of neurons with many responsibilities, one of which is deciding what you should be focusing on.

It also filters out what sensory inputs it believes to be irrelevant so the brain does not have to process more than it can handle. When you vividly imagine specific goals, desires, or tasks, you're effectively giving your brain clarity and direction, communicating to it exactly what you consider to be important, and rehearsing new ways of responding to familiar situations.

Even the act of closing your eyes during a visualization exercise helps with this filtering. About 80 percent of your sensory input comes from sight, so if you close your eyes and go inward, you reduce sensory stimulation, disconnecting from an external world telling you what to do, think, be, or buy and reconnecting with your internal *self*, where your values and beliefs are located. In this state, you can more easily observe the thoughts coming to mind, notice the emotions attached to them, and realize how they're connected to old experiences and states of being. From here, you can imagine how you'd prefer to be and feel, and conjure visions of who you are choosing to become instead.

And these visions can have some major impacts on the way you actually live your life. As you repeatedly visualize these new ways of responding and being, you strengthen the neural pathways associated with them, making them more likely to be activated in real-life situations. This can lead to a shift in automatic responses over time as your brain becomes more accustomed to the new, desired reactions.

Visualizing having done something, whether it's achieving a

goal, attaining a desire, or completing a task, is helpful as a form of mental rehearsal. In fact, as far as the brain is concerned, visualizing yourself doing something is not that far removed from actually *doing* it. The brain struggles to differentiate between reality and imagination. When you worry about a potential situation and imagine every way that things might go wrong, your brain and your body begin to experience stress as if those worst-case scenarios were happening in real life. The opposite is true too, and we can use this to our advantage to help us anticipate positive future outcomes and move forward if we're feeling stuck. Visualizing something going well, using it to mentally rehearse the perfect outcome, and *feeling* the ease can redirect your brain and create confidence over time.

## Let's Meet Your Future Self

Imagine that you're looking at an old photo of yourself as a kid. Even though you know it's you, you might feel like you're looking at a different person because you've changed so much over the years. That's kind of how your brain sees your future self too. When you think about your future self, your brain reacts in a way that's similar to how it would when you think about someone you don't know. This can make it tough to make decisions that benefit your future self because it feels like you're doing things for someone abstract rather than yourself.

The mental movie visualization exercise in the next section will help you not only imagine your future self, but also identify with her. It will help you see your future self in a positive light, and help you step *into* her shoes and see the world through her eyes. The vivid feelings that come from practicing this exercise will let you build a connection with this version of yourself, one that will help you make sacrifices today that will pay off in the long run.

### The Mental Movie Visualization Exercise

It all starts with a dream. A picture in your head of how things *could be*. Possibility. Forward motion. Hope.

As a child, you used your imagination to dream all the time. You dreamed of who you would become when you were older, where you would go, the things you would see, and how you'd spend your money. The world was so big. Your options were endless, infused with hope, fun, and possibility. Even in darker moments of anger and pain, you imagined your future with such promise, intensity, and hope. You knew that one day, you'd be old enough to do what you wanted.

Your imagination may have experienced a few dents, scratches, and falls since childhood. Somewhere along the line, as you entered adulthood and took on its responsibilities, you may have forgotten the truth of possibility, but you *can* always choose again. You can choose again right now.

I know that what I'm saying right now might not match up with the story you've historically told about yourself. Because so many conversations about ADHD center on our struggles, we can start to overidentify with them and see ourselves as problems if we're not careful. We can come to see "distracted" and "lazy" as a normal way of being, and lose all hope of what's possible. It doesn't have to be this way. You can feel better than you ever have before, despite ADHD.

So, what if we start over right now? With a fresh slate, you can give yourself a chance to see yourself differently and give your brain a new blueprint.

There's someone in your future whom you haven't met yet. You'd fall over in (happy!) shock if you met her right now. First, let's release some tension and let the body relax. You can do that by taking a minute to drop out of your thinking brain, and drop into feeling your body by just noticing where you are and what you feel:

- Where in your body do you feel the seat, chair, or earth beneath you? Become aware of the different pressure points.

- What are your elbows touching? Let them be heavy.

- Notice your chest rising and falling.

- Feel your breath as it enters your body and notice where it travels in the body before it leaves again.

- Now, slowly breathe in for four seconds, hold the breath
  for four seconds, and breathe it all out for eight seconds.

Now that you're feeling relaxed and grounded, almost drowsy, close your eyes. Imagine the ultimate future version of yourself who feels her healthiest, happiest self. She's radiant. She's full of love for herself and life.

Where is she?

What is she wearing?

How does she hold herself?

Notice her happiness, her smile, her vibrancy, with curiosity.

Use all your senses to make the visualization as vivid and real as possible. Feel the emotions associated with *being* her. Bring your attention to how it *feels* to be this healthy, happy, joyful. As you visualize your future self in this moment in time, take a photo of it in your mind. Maybe take a photo as she twirls, or as she walks toward you, or as she shows she's alive with energy in the gym. Hold this still frame in your mind.

Now, come back to the present moment. Imagine yourself stepping out of your body and walking to the nearest door. When you walk through that door, see your future self waiting for you on the other side of it. Notice how she smiles at you. Step *into* that body, that future self, as if you're trying on a new outfit. For a moment, actually become her.

Notice how this future version of yourself is dancing around a little bit. Laughing. She's lighthearted. She's in the flow. She feels good. *Look out through her eyes;* see what she sees.

Spend a moment exploring how good this feels.

Now step out of that body and run backward to return to yours. Become again the person who exists right now, where you are. Notice what's different.

Repeat this exchange a few times, running back to your current self faster each time.

Now allow yourself to be still. Close your eyes for a moment. Feel the warm, radiant energy you experienced in the body of future you. Give yourself a hug, gently rubbing up and down your arms. Feel grateful, as if the future has already happened. Set an intention to remember that future self and everything about her, remembering that *she* is *you.*

## WRITE HER DOWN

Words that describe your future self:

_____          _____

_____          _____

_____          _____

_____          _____

_____          _____

Words that describe how it felt to be in her body:

_____          _____

_____          _____

_____          _____

_____          _____

What does she want to thank you for doing every day?

_____          _____

_____          _____

_____          _____

_____          _____

_____          _____

What is she asking you to stop being so hard on yourself about?

_____    _____

_____    _____

_____    _____

_____    _____

_____    _____

What is she most excited for you to feel in the future?

_____    _____

_____    _____

_____    _____

_____    _____

_____    _____

What could you do more of now to become her?

_____    _____

_____    _____

_____    _____

_____    _____

_____    _____

What could you do less of now to become her?

_____     _____

_____     _____

_____     _____

_____     _____

_____     _____

## Be Her Now

After you've made the emotional decision to make a change and have gotten to know your future self, the next step is to think and act differently.

In the past, when you've needed to make a change, you may have spent a lot of time waiting for motivation to strike before getting started. Rather than going to the gym now, you settle on *I'll go to the gym on Monday.* The truth is, motivation often doesn't come first. The best way to build motivation is to do what you don't want to do (which also helps your dopamine reserve). You've probably heard it said a million times before, but just take the first step—and then keep taking steps. Sometimes doing the thing you don't want to do is often the best—perhaps the only—option. In fact, the trust and confidence that slowly build over time from doing these things will be your most reliable source of motivation, especially when you combine it with the identity work you've already done in this chapter.

When I created my vision for how I wanted to feel and look, the intensity of that vision got stronger over time as I began practicing my new habits. I believed in myself more because I was doing something that took me closer to that vision every single day. Keeping the promise that I made to myself showed me how every act of self-care moved me closer to being the woman I wanted to be, the woman I saw during my visualization practices. It wasn't just staring at a vision board, wishing, and hoping that brought it to life; it was the little actions tied to the vision that did. I visualized my future self for two minutes when I woke up instead of reaching for Instagram. I saw the act of dragging myself outside for a ten-minute run as a form of self-care. As I felt myself becoming the version of myself that I had created in my mind, I sometimes found myself not needing to look for motivation at all. Being a person who lived well (even with ADHD) was just who I was and what I did. It became who I was.

**Acting in alignment with your future self doesn't mean putting her on a pedestal.** When you hold something or someone on a pedestal, you create a gap between that thing or person and yourself. Idolizing them or seeing them as perfect can lead you to feel inadequate. Future you isn't above you, she's someone who is already inside you. Future you isn't more perfect than current you. She's human and experiences setbacks too, but she also beats herself up less when she falls off track and therefore she is able to bounce back more quickly.

**If you have spent a lot of time doubting your ability to take action and make changes in your life, the pathways in your brain that reinforce this belief are well worn compared to pathways that help you feel more confident and capable.** If feelings of tension start to creep into the picture, you'll be left trying to figure out *how* this future-you goal will happen. You might feel that you need proof of some kind that change is possible, or old "failures" might come to mind. If that's the case, an unhelpful friend named doubt is entering the picture. Do yourself a favor and let it go.

Some reframes and mindset shifts will help you keep your new beliefs at the forefront of your mind and break in those new pathways just like a new pair of shoes. They will help you dramatically shift the way you carry and talk to yourself, make decisions, and bounce back after encountering an obstacle—all of which will help you build deep trust and confidence in yourself over time.

The fact of the matter is you are human. You're going to slip up. But you interrupt the natural learning process when you make a slipup mean something bad about yourself. For example, you might start today by challenging yourself to commit to one hundred days of running as a way to move toward the future you. Then, on day twenty-one, you trip

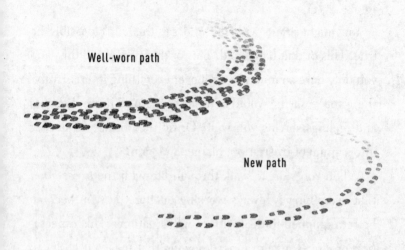

**Well-worn path**

**New path**

over a tree stump. You could make the fall *mean* that you're a clumsy, naturally unfit person and let it be your reason for giving up on becoming fit. Or you could see it for what it is: a mistake that means nothing. You can keep running, or if it no longer feels safe to you, choose another activity by letting your internal GPS do its thing and direct you to something that will help you become the future you.

### Everything Always Works Out for You

You struggle with completing tasks, you don't see projects through, you mess up, you fall down, you get back up again. It can sometimes feel like a never-ending cycle. But what if you approached life as if *everything is always working out for you*?

You might argue with me and say this can't possibly be true. This or that happened. This or that person did this, and you only have so much control over everything in life. Everything you're saying would be valid. But are all those thoughts and feelings serving you well? Or do they bring you deeper into a spiral of frustration, blame, and pain?

When you start to walk through life with the *expectation* that everything is always working out for you, you become better equipped to deal with tough situations. This expectation produces a calm inner knowing that makes it easier to stop sweating the small stuff. When you order something online, you don't sit around worrying about whether it will arrive. You know it will show up exactly as it's meant to, even if you don't know all the steps and the twists and turns your package will take before arriving on your doorstep. Expecting success helps you choose your battles—not everything needs to be a fight to be fought. When things don't go how you expect, you'll have a quiet confidence that you will be okay anyway. When you find a closed door, you're less likely to bang on it, feeling aggravated that it won't open. You might recognize instead that the door could be closed because there is a better one ahead, and you keep moving forward.

Now, this isn't to say we should ignore all discomfort and

feelings of sadness or pain, stuff them down, and avoid feeling them. Doing so will only cause these emotions to accumulate until they overflow and inevitably find their way out. When emotions are ignored, they often intensify. While we may believe we're in control, the truth is that they end up controlling us. But always indulging our emotions after every obstacle can lead to problems.

When you begin recognizing that not all inconveniences are setbacks, you save yourself a lot of unnecessary stress. **These inconveniences might be moments of redirection, and redirection can be a form of protection.** Sometimes it's only in hindsight that we can see we were being led, guided, and protected. Things fade away to make space for what you asked for. Someone or some opportunity leaving your life may be a push forward to meet something that is a better fit, the fit you've asked for. If you are actively and excitedly working toward becoming a future version of yourself, then seeing many elements of your life slowly drifting into the background is actually a *good* sign—it means the process is working. There will be things that need to fall away to make space for the new life you're stepping into.

I often say a belief worth having is a belief worth having, *if the belief is worth having*. So, wouldn't it be worthwhile to believe that ultimately, in the grand scheme of things, *everything is always working out for you*? What if this were so true for you that you started acting and reacting differently, saying no to old habitual thoughts and yes to new ones? What if your future self was so much closer than you think, but the only way to find that out would be to believe it so much that you started *doing* and *being* different, so that future you becomes inevitable?

## THE "APPLY IT TO YOURSELF" RULE

Those of us with ADHD are great at out-of-the-box thinking and problem-solving. We can be great at seeing a silver lining or coming up with a solution to a problem for someone else, but we don't always do that for ourselves. The idea behind the "apply it to yourself" rule is to apply the creative, positive perspective shifts that you suggest to other people to yourself.

I came up with this rule when my partner was traveling for a business retreat. Ruairí was halfway across the world in a hot, normally sunny country when he sent me a photo of a cloudy beach, feeling disappointed about the bad weather. I knew he hadn't taken any sunscreen and probably hadn't bought any yet, so I replied, "That's a pity—maybe it's God protecting you from sunburn before your retreat starts so you don't go in there burned and dehydrated." I was trying to make light of the situation by offering a simple perspective shift to cheer him up about a situation he couldn't control. Then it dawned on me. It was so easy for me to help someone else with a perspective shift, and yet I hadn't been doing that for myself. I'd been beating myself up for forgetting things, making mistakes, and being late, and it was doing nothing but making me feel worse. You cannot plant a flower in a bed of rotten soil and expect it to grow; instead, take care of the soil so the flower can grow.

Now, whenever I run into trouble, I try to remind myself of the way I speak to other people when they're having a hard time— with compassion, with a perspective shift, with *love*. I remind myself of silver linings, and challenge myself to find a bright side, a reason why the situation is working for me, not against me, especially when I can only control my reaction to something and how it affects the rest of my day.

### There Is Evidence You're Already Succeeding

When you assume everything around you is reorganizing and working to make your dream unfold, it becomes easier to notice those coincidences, signs, reminders that you are going to make it. This will give you the nudges you need to keep moving forward. In fact, finding evidence that things are going your way will make the future feel like an imminent possibility rather than an uncertain, distant outcome.

If noticing signs of your success doesn't come naturally to you, try these confidence-boosting practices:

- **Try the "25 good things" gratitude practice:** Instead of writing down just a few things I'm grateful for at the end of the day, I try to find twenty-five and replay them in my mind with my eyes closed. On what first seems like a mundane day, I find myself remembering the cup of tea I enjoyed, the stranger who held the door open for me, or the love I felt while watching my dog run around the park. Take your time and step into the loving emotional state you felt during all these little moments. This practice is especially important on bad, hard, or overwhelming days to remind yourself of the good in your life and that tomorrow will also be filled with little moments of joy. Sometimes I doze off before I get to the twenty-fifth thing, and that's a sure sign of the positive effect the practice has on my nervous system.

- **Decide you'll have a good day:** Right after you wake up, your subconscious mind is most active and soaks up everything, from the thoughts you think to the stuff you hear and what you read, setting the tone for the rest of your day. As soon as you open your eyes, before you even dare think of where you're supposed to go or what the calendar says, try telling yourself, *Today is going to be a great day; It's such a beautiful day; What a day to be alive,* or another variation on this idea. This will direct your mind to find reasons why this is true, create positive expectations for what's ahead, and over time build new neural pathways and reprogram your belief system.

• **Be the person you want to be, right now:** If you were acting as your future self, what would you do? Think about how she would speak to herself, approach challenges, make decisions, and prioritize her time. Then think about how you can start integrating these actions into your present life.

• **Create a happy space:** This can be as simple as a photo album on your phone where you have a bunch of photos of positive experiences you've had. Include moments of achievement when everything worked out, whether it was receiving a diploma, completing a project, or reaching a personal milestone, and moments of personal growth and self-discovery, such as when you tried something new, overcame a challenge, or embraced a self-care practice. Include photos of times when you felt capable, confident; maybe it was a different city or an outfit that helped you feel this way. Add photos of people and pets and places that you're grateful for. Curating this collection of meaningful images will create a visual reminder of the joy, love, and confidence you've experienced in your life, helping you to cultivate an optimistic mindset.

## TRANSFORM INSECURITY INTO EMPOWERMENT

When an old, unhealthy belief comes up, use this exercise to think about how you can replace it instead of trying to force it out of your head. You'll experience less resistance and map a new pathway in your brain.

1. Divide a blank page into two columns. Label one side "Past Self-Beliefs" and the other "Future Self-Beliefs."

2. Under "Past Self-Beliefs," write down all the old beliefs that no longer serve you. Look for beliefs you often think in secret or that contain hints of self-defeat or the victim mentality, such as *The world is against me; I'll be happy when . . .* ; or *I have no control over my life.*

3. Under "Future Self-Beliefs," write down future beliefs that align with health, joy, and abundance, such as *I have the power to change; I was born beautiful, and I am beautiful*; and *I am choosing to be 100 percent responsible for my life.*

4. Use the tips in "Keep Her in Sight, in Mind" on page 89 to keep the new beliefs in the forefront of your mind.

## Remember Her

Your old brain pathways aren't just going to sit there and let you forget about them. They will fight for their survival, pulling you back into your old way of thinking and being. And, of course, you also have ADHD. Remembering new things can be hard, and it's likely you'll forget the woman you saw in your mind's eye, especially if you're going about your everyday life in the same environment where you formed your old beliefs. It's no wonder we forget the goals we set for ourselves and can't think clearly about the future. Just ten minutes of scrolling on social media can overwhelm us with dozens of new pieces of information—and then we overstimulate ourselves further by watching TV at the same time. In our homes, we are surrounded by clutter that screams for our attention. The pile of unread books or the leftovers of the DIY craft session generate silent to-do lists of unfinished tasks. It's so easy to forget that we made a promise to ourselves to be in bed by 11:00 P.M., or to eat a high-protein breakfast, or to meditate for two minutes every morning, or to run a 5K in three months' time.

The only way you're going to feel motivation and take action toward change is if you remember your future self. Remembering her can become a daily practice, and I have a few tricks up my sleeve to help.

### Keep Her in Sight, in Mind

In sight, in mind. If there's one thing you need to remember when it comes to sticking to the goals you've set for yourself, it's this phrase. As someone with ADHD, you need to do everything you can to keep your goals—and the practices that will help those goals happen—as visible as possible.

One solution to this is a visual reminder, which can come in the form of a sticky note or a note card. Whenever I'm going through a period of change and pursuing a new goal or trying to create a new habit, I put sticky notes around my home to remind myself of who I am becoming and to do the things necessary to bring her to life. I place a "TV off at 10:00 P.M." note under my TV, a "Morning sunlight before screen light" note on the wall beside my bed, and a "Protein first" note on my fridge. I tape a little note on my bedroom ceiling or wall so that I'll see it as soon as I wake up. On my bathroom mirror, I keep a note with a line that reminds me to expect the best and helps me shift from an expectation of scarcity to an expectation of abundance. You could also choose to write a few words that describe the healthier, happier version of yourself you're striving to become or the reason for undertaking your new habit.

If sticky notes or note cards won't work for you, type them into your phone's notes app, add them to your phone's and laptop's wallpapers, create a vision board to put next to your bed. Record voice notes to yourself and replay them throughout the day. Make your alarm the sound of your favorite mantra or turn some of your reminders into mantras. You can even use an outfit that you bought for an upcoming event as a visual reminder.

Over time, you may get used to seeing that note card in that exact same spot, making it less noticeable. This is a result of a process called habituation. To help with this, find ways to make it noticeable again: Use a different color of sticky note or note card, move the card, or set an alarm on your phone for the same time every month to check in to see if the visual cue is still working for you.

## THE HEALTHIER, HAPPIER ME IN FIVE WORDS

_____

_____

_____

_____

### Use Audio to Set the Mood

One out-of-the box idea to remind yourself of your vision is to record audio clips of yourself giving uplifting mini pep talks to yourself. Record yourself describing your perfect day, your daily routine, or your new, healthier ways of thinking and being a year from now. Once you've made your recordings, listen to them every morning, or whenever you need an encouraging boost. This is something I started doing many years ago. While it felt silly at first, I noticed that the more I listened to my recordings, the easier it was for me to truly believe both in myself and in the promise of better days ahead.

Another way to use audio to your advantage is through music. A 2022 study showed that listening to music can modulate brain activity, enhance neural connectivity, and promote positive changes in brain function. Associating our future self with music is one of the best ways to remember her, because it can bring up the emotions that we'll experience when we become her. This makes it easier to act in alignment with who we want to become. Another way to use music is to create private playlists that remind you of your goals. For example, I have a collection of songs that make me feel like I'm standing in New York City with my book. I get so excited listening to the songs while imagining myself walking down the street, alive with possibility. It's a total energy changer and lifts my mood!

### Feel Forward

The commitment to create a better life is an ongoing process. You don't just stop brushing your teeth one day because you feel they are clean enough and that should do you for the rest of your life. Your way of looking at your well-being needs to be the same. You don't just stop your healthy habits forever after you've lost those ten pounds or hit that personal best in the marathon or finally established a solid sleep routine. You know that you still have to tend to yourself every day, in whatever way you can on that particular day, while being grateful for where you're at and excited by where you're going.

And, of course, like any process, the road to change is not a linear one. You *will* have setbacks. You *will* have days when you choose the couch over the gym, or your phone over a meditation session. When I feel discouraged, I feel forward. This is my phrase for asking my future self for guidance, as if she's an older sister looking back and cheering me on. I acknowledge the old beliefs coming up and doing what they've always done, but I also look ahead to where I'm going and who I'm choosing to become.

If you're having a hard day, know that your future self is looking back at you, smiling, asking you to be kind and gentle because your success is inevitable. No matter how frustrated you get, or how many times you forget her and fall off course, everything is going to be okay. All your efforts are adding up, and the down days are the parts of the learning curve when you get to know and understand yourself better. You're still learning and embracing the fact that it's safe to change, to move forward, and to choose something different. You're unraveling and releasing decades of harboring old thought patterns, beliefs, and habits. You're getting to know yourself again, you're tuning in to your own innate wisdom and reconnecting with your body. Have patience. You're doing your best. All is well, just keep moving forward.

**Q:** I'm finding it hard to imagine a brighter future. All I see is bad stuff ahead. Is there another way to start changing my beliefs about the future?

**A:** The visualizations you'll need for identity work can be hard to create when you're in a pit of anxiety, fear, and hopelessness. If you find visualizing your future self too much of a stretch, try to envision a better day in your current life, maybe even an ideal day. Visualizing a better day can be easier because it's grounded in familiar routines and experiences, whereas imagining a potential future, which comes with changes and uncertainties, might bring on feelings of anxiety.

Imagine going for a walk and noticing the sun briefly peeking through the clouds and feeling its warmth on your face. Maybe you're on your way to your favorite bookshop, café, or park. Maybe your schedule is free because someone said they'd take care of everything else. Maybe your phone is set on airplane mode. You feel peaceful, in the flow, unhurried and relaxed. You feel so calm, you're even smiling at strangers passing you by. Maybe you have new habits and are starting to notice that glow a little more. It's subtle, but you see it and feel it. You feel proud of yourself for taking little steps forward. Even though it's hard, you said yes to a healthier, happier you and you're glad you did. Imagine this person in as much detail as possible until you feel something, and then, as you move through your day, remember her.

# 4

###### ■

# Move More

*Movement is medicine.*

When I'm feeling irritable, restless, anxious, on edge, I picture a frayed shoelace. It's what I imagine the inside of every cell in my brain looks like when I am feeling *off*. Even my partner, Ruairí, knows about the shoelace. "I need to fix the shoelace" is all I need to say to explain how I'm feeling and what I need to do: move.

A few minutes into a run, I see this shoelace transform in my mind. The frayed edges tighten and zip up as I'm moving. I even hear a *ding!* in my mind as the shoelace completes this little transformation. My brain is working again. I remember who I am and what makes me feel like *me*. My body was craving movement, and with movement, I've released some stress.

## IS IT ANXIETY, OR IS YOUR BODY BEGGING FOR MOVEMENT?

By the time I was diagnosed with ADHD, I had reached a really low point—I was desperate for change, and now that I had a diagnosis, I *needed* to find a way to manage my ADHD better. After doing a deep dive into the research, I quickly realized that exercise is one of the most effective nonpharmaceutical treatments for ADHD. Think of it this way: Adderall, one of the most popular medications for ADHD treatment, and similar stimulants improve focus and reduce impulsivity by increasing dopamine and norepinephrine levels in the brain. You know what else increases dopamine and norepinephrine levels? Exercise.

Instead of exercising three or four times a week for an hour in the gym like I'd always done, I started exercising daily for shorter bursts of time to help manage my overactive ADHD brain and the anxiety and emotional dysregulation I was experiencing due to worsening executive dysfunction. Tightening the shoelace is my visual metaphor for using movement to ease that anxious, buzzy feeling so many of us experience when our ADHD symptoms flare up.

People have this idea that ADHD looks like an eight-year-old boy running and jumping across the room. But for many women, hyperactivity is often internal and manifests as anxiety and all the things that come along with feeling anxious.

Unlike the hyperactive little boy bouncing around, most of your movements are happening in your brain. Your racing, unorganized thoughts jump from one topic to another, and you mix in feelings of judgment and worry. You feel like you have a browser window with ten tabs open as you're thinking about all the things you need to do—or should be doing.

**You can't think your way out of this extra internal energy; you have to move it out.** We need to move to tighten up that shoelace and find an outlet for it before it spirals out of control.

But you don't need to wait until the point of a panic attack to utilize the power of exercise. In fact, our bodies will always let us know that they need to move by sending distress signals in the form of irritability or restlessness, which we might interpret as anxiety. When I let these signals linger for too long, I begin to experience heightened forms of psychological distress such as trypophobia, the fear of patterns of holes. It's a sign that I'm not moving the extra energy out of my body, allowing my mind to use it to create threats, even if these threats aren't real. If I don't take this distress signal seriously and move more, it can lead to debilitating anxiety and overwhelm.

Of course, moving every day can be a challenge if you have ADHD, because we struggle with organization and creating structure in our daily lives. But remember the vicious cycle described on page 4. Not moving can make us feel worse. Movement is part of life. We are built to move, to be agile, and to feel alive. Yes, I know it's hard to get up and go and do it, but we can train ourselves to burn off that energy and to know how good it's going to feel afterward. And knowing how good it feels afterward is what motivates us to do it again, to *keep moving*.

*Movement is part of life. We are built to move,*
*to be agile, and to feel alive.*

## Why Movement Matters

- **It increases blood flow to the brain:** Exercise increases blood flow to the brain, which is crucial for its proper functioning. When blood flow is low in the prefrontal cortex—the part of the brain responsible for attention, impulse control, and organization—ADHD symptoms can worsen. However, better blood flow provides the necessary oxygen and nutrients for the brain to work efficiently. This allows us to think more clearly, make better decisions, and better regulate our emotions and behavior.

- **It promotes the growth of new brain cells:** Movement sparks your body's production of brain-derived neurotrophic factor and other proteins that promote the growth of new neurons in the brain. In the past, it was believed that the adult brain couldn't grow new neurons, but we now understand that the brain has the ability to generate these important cells throughout life. In fact, it's been found that humans can create new brain cells into their nineties. Neurons send and receive messages throughout the brain and body to help you think, feel, and move. With movement, you create more of these little messengers to make your brain work better, just as adding more workers to a team will get things done faster and more smoothly. As a result, you experience improved focus, learning, memory, mood regulation, stress resilience, and flexibility in thinking.

- **It releases feel-good neurotransmitters**: Exercise not only helps your brain make new cells, it also triggers the release of feel-good neurotransmitters such as dopamine, serotonin, and oxytocin. These neurotransmitters are often called "happy hormones" because they help regulate your emotions. Even just a few minutes of movement can lead to the release of these neurotransmitters, which can improve mood and attention and leave you feeling more focused, energized, and in control. So when you move your body, you're not just exercising—you're giving your brain a powerful boost too!

- **It rewires your brain's reward system**: Habits such as daily movement can change the structure and function of the brain's reward circuitry by increasing dopamine levels, the availability of dopamine receptors, their sensitivity to dopamine, and protection against dopamine depletion. It also changes how the brain cells involved in your reward system communicate with one another. Finding a form of movement that you enjoy can make your reward system more responsive, which means your brain gets better at enjoying activities that make you feel good. You can change and enhance your brain! You're not stuck with the model you originally got.

## WHAT YOUR NON-ADHD PERSONAL TRAINER DIDN'T TELL YOU ABOUT EXERCISE

I've worked with thousands of women over the last decade, and based on that experience I think it's safe to say you know exercise is good for you, and that you're not doing enough of it.

*"Lisa, if I was able to find the energy to go to the gym, I'd be doing it! I don't want to work out. I can't stick to anything, I find it boring, the gym scares me, everyone looks at me, and I don't know what to do."*

Trust me, I hear you. ADHD gets in the way, especially when executive dysfunction takes control. **I find that executive dysfunction is one of the biggest barriers we face** when it comes to exercising and other healthy habits because it distracts us from the relief that exercise can bring. Usually the exercise itself isn't the problem. It's the steps that lead up to moving that make us feel stuck or overwhelmed: choosing what exercise to do, changing into workout clothes, getting ourselves out the door to travel to where we will exercise. Sometimes we just forget to go to the gym or to bring our running shoes. We forget that exercise can help us feel calmer, and that we even have a goal to move more. While some people can navigate all these steps on autopilot, we have to coach ourselves through each step and be cautious not to fall prey to the distractions that can derail us between these steps.

This is the very reason we need to approach exercise differently. We're not lazy or unmotivated. Sometimes the idea of a long workout in the gym feels too overwhelming, and it's easier to stay home. Our brains have problems creating and keeping up with routines, but the good news is that exercise doesn't have to look like going to the gym for an hour and following the exact workout your trainer laid out for you or doing what you see on social media. It can be easy. It can be intuitive.

## You Can Learn to Love Exercise

Gyms can be so intimidating, and I say this as someone who's been a fitness trainer for more than a decade. When I walk into a new gym, I still feel awkward and out of place until I get to know the space. It brings back memories of when I first started using gyms as a teenager. The machines looked terrifying. I didn't want to try using one in case I did something wrong and everyone stared at me, so I stuck to the treadmill or cross trainer.

I've spoken to many clients who have similarly negative associations with exercise. They dreaded the idea of starting an exercise routine. They had a bad experience at a gym, with a trainer, or during a PE class as a child, or they feel awkward as a beginner in a new space. They often tell me something I've heard way too often: "I hate exercise."

Do you hate exercise, or do you hate the way you were shown to exercise? Here's the thing: Identifying as someone who hates exercise—and doesn't do it—keeps you stuck in a negative feedback loop. You can't know how good exercise feels until you're in the middle of doing it. But because you identify as someone who hates to exercise, you never do it, so you keep identifying as someone who hates it. And because behavior almost always matches identity, you deprive yourself of the opportunity to find out how good it feels.

*Do you hate exercise, or do you hate the way you were shown to exercise?*

By saying "I hate exercise," you've put an endless universe of ways to exercise into one teeny, tiny box that you won't touch. At some point, you'll need to open this box if you want to soak up the benefits of moving more. When you challenge that identity-forming belief, the belief might rise to the surface, offering you the opportunity for transformation beyond your wildest dreams.

This was what happened to me with running. I was someone who said she didn't run. I would tell people "I hate running," and because I hated running, I never ran. I admired runners but *insisted* I could never be one. Then one of my friends decided to complete a hundred-day running challenge. She posted daily selfies on Instagram for accountability. I noticed she was holding herself differently. Her energy was magnetic and confident. It was undeniable—something about my friend's daily runs was resonating with me.

One sunny morning, I felt inspired to wake up my brain and took a baby step. I decided to go for a quick run, and afterward, I tagged my friend, thanking her for the inspo.

She messaged me back: "You do know you now have to run for 100 days, right? You have to do it."

My initial reaction? "Eh, no."

But curiosity lingered. I asked her how she felt after a hundred days. She told me she was able to problem-solve while running, and that she felt more creative than ever. The first thirty days weren't enjoyable, but after day sixty, she said, she craved her runs and looked for more challenging routes.

By day one hundred, my friend said she felt incredible. Life felt smoother because of these runs. She was healthier than ever—that was made clear by the way she was glowing.

Still, I didn't want to do it. Though I had made the small shift from "I never run" to "I'll run sometimes, but not every day," my belief that I wasn't a runner still had a hold over me. I couldn't commit to running a hundred days in a row because *I was not a runner and I hated running*.

Deep down inside, I knew what was really happening. I had closed myself to the possibility of changing my ways. When I realized this, I went for another run, and even though I felt terribly unfit at first—I was out of breath and had to stop every twenty seconds to rest—I was on top of the world when I finished my route around the forest. I felt like that future self I saw in my visualization practices. I was able to remember her more easily, and I experienced a surge of belief, trust, and faith that my transformation into the healthier, happier version of myself was not just possible, but inevitable. I wanted to hold on to this feeling forever, and in that moment I promised myself more of it. So there I was, all in for one hundred days of running, as a lifelong nonrunner who couldn't jog the length of herself.

One day while in the middle of a run, I realized that running wasn't the problem. The thing I disliked was my rules around what running should look like. I realized that I didn't need to do a couch to 5K. I didn't need to run without stopping. I didn't have to stick to a running program. I could run for the length of one song and go home again, and I could stop and start as often as I wanted to.

This one small recognition was a huge catalyst for transformation. It created a domino effect that helped me explore other healthy habits. It felt empowering to take an old, limiting belief and break it in half. The experience reminded me that there's so much possibility and potential beyond the assumptions we hold about ourselves. I didn't need to be athletic to run, but I could choose to become an athletic person by running if I wanted to.

---

*There's so much possibility and potential beyond the assumptions we hold about ourselves.*

---

## REWRITE YOUR EXERCISE STORY

If you want to drop the "I hate exercise" piece of your identity and become someone who moves more, a great way to start is to simply tap into your curiosity:

- What are you gaining by not exercising? Or by being someone who hates all exercise and holding on to that identity?

- Do you really hate *all* gyms, classes, and trainers? Are you really hopeless or a lost cause, unable to find any way of moving that you enjoy?

- What stories do you tell about exercise? Can you consider letting them go?

- What memories do you have of feeling emotional discomfort while exercising? Did you feel forced to exercise in ways you didn't enjoy when you were younger?

- Has exercise always been tied to the idea that you only do it to lose weight or to punish yourself for eating?

- Have your exercise choices always been high intensity, leaving you exhausted and out of breath?

If you uncover a lot of negative attitudes about exercise, it's no surprise you don't like it! If this is you, the next section will help you discover new and exciting ways to move. It's possible to find a low-impact, calming, grounding movement practice that doesn't leave you exhausted and frustrated. Once you do, it has the potential to change your life.

If you aren't feeling open to the possibility of changing this mindset, I urge you to return to chapter 3 and review the foundations of identity work. Without a compelling vision of what's possible, it's too easy to give in to the lie that you are trapped as you are, unable to change. I don't want you to go running every day just for the sake of running. I want you to have a lifestyle shift, an identity shift. You are becoming a healthy, fit person. You are someone who loves moving in some way every day because it helps you feel so much healthier and happier, and because it's a great way to help you manage your ADHD.

## You Can Swap Workouts for Movement

When studying the Blue Zones, the places in the world where people live the longest, the journalist Dan Buettner found that one key commonality shared by the people who lived there was daily movement. Notice I didn't use the word "exercise." In fact, many of the people in these areas didn't consider their daily movement to be exercise at all.

Whether they were getting their heart rate up by gardening or walking around their hilly neighborhood, they regularly engaged in activities that required them to be active. When they left their homes, they chose to walk to wherever they were going. Many of them moved their body every twenty minutes or so just by going about their day. Instead of setting aside time to exercise, the people who live the longest have daily movement effortlessly baked into their lifestyle. It isn't something they think about doing; it's just something they *do*. It's who they are. It's part of their identity. It isn't something extra to check off on a to-do list.

In other words, moving—and all the good that comes from it—doesn't have to be a big deal.

**When I started seeing exercise as a tool to manage my ADHD, I was still holding on to the narrative telling me that there needed to be rules and goals with each workout for it to "matter."** These old restrictions were still haunting me. And the negative beliefs they reinforced became crippling when they joined forces with executive dysfunction. Thoughts like *I need to run for thirty minutes* or *I need to get ready to follow this exact program* would make movement feel so daunting it would put me off doing anything at all.

When I started my hundred-day running challenge, I set this intention: All I needed to do was to simply run for a hundred days in a row. That's it. I didn't care about distance, time, schedule, or speed. It didn't matter what time of day I ran. It didn't matter what distance I ran, or how long I ran for. I wasn't comparing current runs with old runs or measuring myself against anyone else. I wasn't going to track how fast I could run a 5K without stopping because at that point, I

couldn't run a 5K without stopping.* I didn't pressure myself
to run the whole time while I was out. It didn't matter if I ran
for forty seconds and then needed to walk a bit until I could
run again. I listened to my body, alternating between running
and walking until I wanted to go home. The point was that I
was running. All that mattered was that I was cementing in a
daily habit by consciously *choosing* to put on my running
shoes and get out the door. That image in my mind and that
simple intention were what kept me motivated and helped
make the challenge enjoyable.

Still, not every day came naturally. On day seventy-six, it was
almost bedtime when I realized I hadn't done my run. There
were plenty of streetlights on, so I felt safe enough to go outside and get it done—even if it was just a quick one. I popped
my workout clothes on, went out in the dark, and ran up and
down my street for literally two and a half minutes while Ruairí
watched me from the window. I put no pressure on myself to
go beyond that. I just needed to get on my shoes, run a little,
hear the bell ding in my mind, and feel proud of myself for
continuing the hundred-day streak. It was like a game to me.

By redefining exercise as movement, I gave myself the
opportunity to see and feel myself winning the battle

---

* To be honest, I still don't know if I can run a 5K without stopping because that was never a goal.

against the executive-dysfunction demon. Forgetting to go on my run was no longer a roadblock that stopped me in my tracks, but rather something I could easily navigate around without getting angry at myself for forgetting.

There are endless ways to move. If you're trying something new or something you haven't done for a while, you'll probably feel off-balance, heavy, uncoordinated, and a bit awkward, but you'll also *start to feel good*.

After just a few minutes at it, your choice of outfit won't matter. What people are thinking won't matter. The time of day won't matter. The negative memory that you've held on to won't matter. You'll hit the sweet spot. Trust me. That sweet spot is what you need to use as your anchor. Savor that feeling when you get it; close your eyes and enjoy it.

### What Type of Movement Should I Choose?

Because people are excited by different things during different times in life, I'm not going to give you a set program that tells you the exact workouts you must do a certain number of days a week. What I want to give you instead is a set of criteria you can come back to as your interests change so you can naturally progress to whatever else catches your interest. When it's time to choose how to move your body, I suggest you begin with something that:

- gets your heart rate up

- feels like a challenge

- stimulates sweating

- allows for flexibility in the approach

- can be done every day for the length of at least one song (a few minutes)

- gets you out of your thinking head and into the present moment

If you want a more specific place to start or ideas for types of movement you can do at a gym, here are my top recommendations to weave into your sessions:

- **Unilateral movements:** Unilateral movements are exercises that focus on working one side of the body at a time rather than both sides. These exercises challenge stability, coordination, and balance because they require the body to stabilize itself while performing the movements. This promotes focus and coordination and helps you practice bringing your attention to the here and now and develop a deeper connection between the mind and body. Examples of unilateral movements are single-arm kettlebell swings, side planks, single-leg presses, and single-leg hops.

- **Giant sets:** Giant sets are when you perform multiple exercises back-to-back with little to no rest in between. Unlike supersets, which typically involve two exercises, giant sets involve three or more exercises targeting the same muscle group or related muscle groups. They're great for pushing past workout plateaus, boosting how long your muscles can keep going, and making your workouts more interesting by mixing things up. Giant sets are beneficial for ADHD brains and executive dysfunction. They have a simple setup, so there's less need to make decisions during your workout or to walk around the gym looking for the next thing to do. The rapid transitions between exercises help keep your mind engaged and prevent boredom or distraction. You can just grab a kettlebell, go to a corner of the gym, and pick four or more moves to do consecutively without stopping.

- **Proprioceptive exercises:** Proprioceptive exercises are activities that aim to improve the body's ability to sense its position, movement, and actions, and focus on enhancing awareness of body position, coordination, balance, and control, which are often areas of difficulty for those of us with ADHD. Proprioceptive moves can also regulate your nervous system (we'll talk about the importance of a regulated nervous system in chapter 8), helping you feel calmer and more grounded. Examples of proprioceptive exercises include activities that involve pushing, pulling, or squeezing, as well as ones that challenge balance and coordination, such as yoga or martial arts. For example, you could practice push-ups on an unstable surface such as a balance pad or wobble board to challenge stability.

- **Racket sports:** Racket sports like ping-pong, pickleball, padel, and tennis offer significant benefits due to their dynamic nature, which helps release excess energy and enhance focus and attention. These sports require hand-eye coordination, timing, and quick reflexes, leading to improvements in motor skills, spatial awareness, and mental alertness. Despite involving dynamic movement and rapid changes in direction, racket sports are generally low-impact activities, making them suitable for various fitness levels. Pickleball and similar racket sports provide a workout for the brain, stimulating both the cerebellum with their fast pace and the frontal lobes with the strategy involved, and promoting overall brain health and function. Numerous activities can produce health and longevity benefits, but racket sports consistently rank as the best sports for promoting a longer life. A study of more than eight thousand people over twenty-five years found that those who played tennis lived nearly *ten years* longer.

What about HIIT (high-intensity interval training)? That typically involves rapid, repetitive movements or exercises performed at maximum effort, such as sprinting or doing jumping jacks or burpees. For someone with ADHD who may already struggle with fatigue and feeling frazzled, HIIT may feel overwhelming and exhausting and just increase your stress level, especially during times when your energy is naturally lower throughout the month, such as during the luteal phase of your menstrual cycle (starting around two weeks before your period starts and ending when you get your period). Instead of forcing yourself through a forty-five-minute HITT class that adds to your overwhelm, prioritize low-impact exercises that provide a sense of calm, such as Pilates, vinyasa yoga, or proprioceptive exercises that focus on improving body awareness, control, and alignment. If you're craving movement with high intensity to elevate your heart and breathing rates, scatter bouts of high-intensity activity throughout your low-intensity workout. For example, you can do a minute of fast skipping, burpees, or sprints after every ten-minute Pilates sequence.

### Feel Free to "Fail"

In my midtwenties, I used bodybuilding competitions to get in shape and stay on track. I loved the challenge of these competitions, but when it came to my goals, the effects were never consistent. I would gain back any weight I had lost in training once the competition was completed, and because I didn't do the identity work needed to support these changes, I always felt like I was failing. The overfamiliarity of bodybuilding also left me stuck. While I got a thrill from the challenge of competing and this kept me motivated to go to the gym, it wasn't a sustainable way of motivating myself.

Still, bodybuilding was what I was used to. After experiencing cycles of burnout in 2016, I left my home and life in Ireland to work online as a digital nomad, starting in Dubai, then making my way to Thailand, until I eventually settled in London (more about burnout in chapter 8). While I was in Dubai, I sought out an in-demand personal trainer who had prepped many people for bodybuilding shows through his online program. I paid for his service and waited for my program to come by email. I was so excited about getting the results I wanted—less body fat, visible abs, and the feeling of being fit and athletic.

I followed his instructions precisely. I went to the gym four days a week and took rest days in between. The first batch of workouts was fine because the exercises were new to me and

I was excited to get started, but I quickly got bored of doing the same ones on repeat each week. Hearing the words "progressive overload" was enough to put me to sleep. I wanted to jump, spin, run, and dance, but I felt like I had to stick with this program because I genuinely believed it was the only way to meet my goals. Besides, I was so sore on the rest days that I didn't even have the energy to add in the types of movement my body was craving.

I then spent two weeks in Bali teaching at a health-and-wellness retreat. I adored the freedom of listening to my body again, honoring its ebbs and flows. After the retreat, I never emailed my trainer for my weekly check-ins again. At the time, I felt a bit embarrassed that I couldn't seem to stick to his program for the prescribed twelve weeks, but I also felt free. Structured bodybuilding-style weight-lifting programs were what I knew best for years. I had always dabbled in yoga, running, Pilates, and many other forms of exercise, but at that time I had this inflexible mindset that told me that heavy weights were what was right, and that I had to stick to that and take rest days in between—even if that routine wasn't doing it for me anymore.

In hindsight, I know it wasn't that the trainer couldn't help me. He simply wasn't the coach for me. I didn't fail, and he didn't fail. As someone with ADHD, I needed something interactive, flexible, exciting, and challenging to keep me engaged in my workouts. I started realizing that shorter bursts of movement each day work better for my ADHD brain than longer workouts a couple of times per week.

**I must stick to this twelve-week program. ➔ I can move in whatever way I want to today.**

When you feel unable to stick to advice or programs and get frustrated, it might be because the advice is coming from coaches and trainers who don't understand the ADHD brain or the female body. It might not be you, but rather the people you're listening to. I know your personal trainer, fitness book, or program might have told you that there's a "right" way to work out: *You must stick to this program this many days a week. You must lift this many pounds. You must do barbell squats. You must log it all.* I used to be that girl who listened to the personal trainer, and I used to *be* that personal trainer. But now I'm here to tell you that you don't have to do any of this if you don't want to.

**What's right is what currently interests you, today. Not what Ben Bro PT tells you is right.**

It doesn't matter how correct the personal trainer is in terms of programming and science; if you find your exercise routine boring, you're not going to get results, because you're not going to do it, full stop. There might be seasons when the training regimen from Ben Bro PT is exactly what you need, and in those seasons it will serve you well. If that's you right now, great, keep it up! But know that when you get bored, it's okay to switch to something else. And when you're over-whelmed, it's okay to switch to something smaller, easier, with fewer rules. I want you to do what works for you today. Sometimes that looks completely different from what every-body else in the gym is doing. And that's okay.

You're not failing. You're changing your mind.

---

*I want you to do what works for you today. Sometimes that looks completely different from what everybody else in the gym is doing. And that's okay.*

---

Our culture often confuses changing your mind with fail-ure, but not sticking to one thing isn't a blemish on your char-acter, nor does it say anything about you as a human. There is no shame in trying out running and stopping after a few weeks to take up tennis. Or stopping tennis to sign up for a month of yoga. Or getting bored with that and giving Cross-Fit a try for a year. You're still moving and getting fit. And if you ask me, **trying different things is a sign that you're curious, resourceful, and capable of change when some-thing isn't working.** Being a person who is willing to be a beginner over and over again screams confidence.

Sure, if you'd stayed with running you might have become a running coach by now, but that wasn't what you wanted. Again, your goal is to become the healthiest, happiest version of yourself, and shaming yourself for changing or internalizing shaming statements from the people around you doesn't need to get in your way.

I can't stick to anything. → I get to experience so much of the world.

| PROGRESS | ALSO PROGRESS |
|---|---|
| △ △ △ △ △ | △ △ △ ○ ○ |
| △ △ △ △ △ | ○ ○ ○ ○ □ |
| △ △ △ △ △ | □ □ △ △ △ |
| △  Running | △  Running |
|  | ○  Tennis |
|  | □  CrossFit |

## HOW TO MOVE (ALMOST) EVERY DAY

If you are open to committing to moving regularly as part of who you are and who you are choosing to become, I invite you to explore and allow yourself to be open to the different ways you want to move in. The options that work for your body and lifestyle are limitless when movement can look however you want it to. Maybe you're someone who loves playing tennis and has easy access to a court. Maybe you're someone who loves boxing. Maybe you're someone who loves swimming. Skipping rope in your backyard might be a good idea. Think back to the Blue Zones—maybe you live in a hilly area and moving is as simple as opting for a daily uphill walk first thing in the morning.

Once you pick the types of movement you'd like to try, read on to see how you can make them a habit.

## Find Excitement in the Process

What excited me about my hundred-days-of-running challenge wasn't the running, but rather the idea of forming a new habit and the game of maintaining my movement streak. In other words, I was excited by the *process*. Simply continuing my streak gave me the feeling that I was accomplishing something. It activated reward pathways in my brain that made me want to run the next day.

You can do the same with your favorite form of movement. **Instead of waiting until you lose weight or build muscle to feel like you've reached a goal, treat the process of movement as its own reward.** Every day you move, you'll recondition your mind and your body. This hack also helps you stay present instead of being constantly en route to a destination that feels far away. You'll feel that you've arrived by finding enjoyment in the daily movement, trusting that it is now all working out for you, taking your time, and knowing that eventually you'll turn your visualizations into reality.

## Keep Yourself Guessing

With ADHD, we need to be super intentional about the way we go about conquering a new challenge. Eventually, a wave of boredom will wash over us when the novelty wears off, urging us to throw in the towel and making it tough to find motivation.

When I'm feeling unmotivated, I've learned from past experience that to reset my motivation, I need to do something challenging or uncomfortable (but safe) instead of waiting for motivation to magically appear. This helps trigger the release of dopamine in a healthy way, which essentially teaches me that there's a reward in doing the hard thing I'm avoiding.

In other words, support the health of your dopamine system, play a dopamine game (see page 28), and do something you don't want to do. Once in a while, drag yourself out of bed at sunrise to go for a run *when that's the last thing you want to do* and have a coffee at your favorite café afterward (but only if you do the sunrise run).

Let me make this clear: You don't need to force yourself to do really hard things all the time. Doing this every day can make you resent the act of moving at all, and you'll just stop. But giving yourself these (annoying) challenges now and again will boost your motivation and improve your brain health in the long term. **When more effort is needed to get pleasure, your brain grows.**

While you don't want to do the really hard thing every day, there are still ways to keep your workout routine interesting on a more daily basis. For example, what helped keep my runs interesting was to approach some of them with a spirit of adventure. I would try different paths, trails, and parks. I tested how it would feel to run at different times of day. I ran while I was fasting and during times when I wasn't.

As I experimented, I always took notice of how I felt and enjoyed the fact that I was learning so much more about myself. I used the Strava app to hold myself accountable and enjoyed the surge of excitement when I got to click that "complete" button and name each run Day 17, Day 18, and so on. (I kept my settings private for safety.)

Novelty is key for the ADHD brain to sustain excitement and motivation. If you start feeling reluctant to move on a regular basis, it might be time to make a more drastic change. Maybe you need to switch gyms, find a new running buddy, or swap the training PDF at home for a studio that offers you a chance to join an in-person community.

## FINDING A GYM THAT YOU LOVE

A quarter of the way into my hundred-days-of-running challenge, I started craving other ways of moving again—weight lifting, yoga, Pilates, and boot-camp classes. I went to try out a local gym in the area of London that my partner and I had recently moved to. After paying for two day passes, I had already started to dread going. I didn't like the layout. It was too bright, busy, and crowded. I knew it wasn't the right one for me, and there was no way I would keep going to it.

I soon found one I absolutely loved. There was so much space, with numerous empty rooms and options for different classes. I also just loved the vibe. I felt like the best version of myself walking into that gym. I loved how I felt in that building, and that feeling made me excited to be there.

We need to choose our gyms like we choose our life partners—with standards, a feeling of joy and excitement, and love. You won't want to check out of a great relationship, and you won't want to check out of a great gym or studio. So don't settle. Make sure your gym is a place that you enjoy and you're truly excited about. Environment matters, especially to someone with ADHD. Here are some features that make a gym space ADHD-friendly:

- An open space with many different rooms, nooks, and corners where you can go to be alone and do your own thing if you want to avoid the crowded areas.

- Music that isn't so loud it overpowers your headphones and causes sensory overload.

- Natural lighting from windows; if the gym doesn't have natural lighting, I find moodier lighting is better than clinically bright ceiling lights.

- A schedule of different types of classes for when you need novelty.

- A sense of safety. It's important to feel safe in a space if you want to keep coming back to it. Without it, you'll find ways to avoid going.

- A sauna (or another interesting feature) for low-motivation days. When I really lack motivation, I go to the gym just to use the sauna and always end up moving a little bit while I'm passing the stretching area.

If you live in a remote part of the world without accessible options, your challenge is to find an online platform or trainer you love and create a small space for yourself somewhere at home. Your sacred space to move would ideally be as distraction-free as possible. I keep a mini trampoline in the corner of my living room, and I use it regularly to shake off stressful energy, move my lymphatic system, and keep myself energized between solo work and meetings.

## Apply the Right Type of Pressure

When boredom strikes and saps our motivation, we can work through these feelings by applying just the right amount of pressure on ourselves. This requires a delicate balance—**too much pressure can put us into a state of paralysis and overwhelm, yet not enough of it can leave us bored and forgetting about our goals altogether.** We have to stretch a little beyond our comfort zone, but not too far. Tasks that are too easy might not stimulate the brain, but tasks that are too difficult can lead to frustration, and eventually to throwing in the towel. Finding a balance between effort and enjoyment is important for promoting neuroplasticity.

Knowing this, I avoided placing too many guidelines on my running challenge. If I had insisted on running a 5K every day for my run to "count," I would have absolutely stopped on day three from exhaustion. As I mentioned earlier, by giving myself **flexibility** and setting the **intention** of just running every day, I could focus on enjoying the challenge and taking it one day at a time.

On the days when I couldn't be bothered to go outside, I put the pressure back on by returning to identity work and keeping sight of my future self. I chose to *remember her,* to remember my future self, who had completed this challenge. I would close my eyes and create a movie scene in my mind of *having done it.* Viewing this scene let me experience what it would feel like to complete the challenge. I'd see myself slowing down my run to finish, smiling widely, and I'd notice the *feeling* of relief in my body. Seeing all that I dream of, alive in my mind, is the most therapeutic and motivating activity. These positive feelings are super important. When you associate them with the thing you're avoiding, you can use them to override procrastination and avoidance. They made it easier to remember why I said yes to the challenge in the first place.

## Visualize While You're Moving

I use visualization not only as a source of motivation for moving, I also use it while I'm in motion. I imagine my future self in different situations. I see her running on the beach. I see her laughing. I see her in the gym, walking around her home office, writing her next book. I notice what she's wearing, her energy, how fit and healthy she is. I keep seeing until I feel something and then I really tap into the *feeling*.

The next time you feel really challenged as you're moving, all you need to do is use your big, beautiful imagination. Bring the image of your future self into your mind and breathe some life into it. Know you are bringing this version of yourself to life in this very moment with the exact thing that you are doing right now. All of these days, all of these habits— they add up to this future version of you. Focus on the connection between your imagination and the muscles you're moving. Be present in your body—*feel the change as you move*. Familiarize yourself with how it feels to be at the finish line of your goal, to be living and moving as your future self. Experience the energy boost and happy hormones you're getting from your workout and hit the "save" button in your brain so you can come back to these feelings every time movement feels too hard.

To take this one step further, pair positive statements with movement to help strengthen habit formation. When you repeat these statements while you're in motion, you strengthen the association between the activity and a positive outcome, making it more likely for movement to become a habit and promoting huge, holistic changes in brain function. This approach supports the brain's natural plasticity to create behavior change and an overall positive transformation. You'll start to associate moving with feeling good, and eventually you'll crave it. If you want to really amplify the benefits, add emotion to your words. The next time you move, try saying aloud, "I am fit! I am healthy! I love how I feel when I move!"

If this feels icky, know that the key is *how* you tell yourself. Daily affirmations can be ineffective for many people with low self-esteem. For instance, if you're trying to lose weight but keep saying "I am at my healthy weight," it could cause some friction. Instead, choose a phrase that feels good to you, like "I'm excited to feel fitter and healthier every day." It's important to pick a phrase that feels true to you and still helps you move in the direction you want to go.

## Remove the Obstacles to Starting

Exercise doesn't need all the bells and whistles we often convince ourselves it must have. Allow yourself the freedom of just moving and being without feeling everything needs to be perfect before you start. Remember, we don't give in to the all-or-nothing mentality with *Healthy Happy ADHD*. We value freedom, flexibility, convenience, and ease. **Make it easy! Seize the easy!** Let's remove the mental clutter and streamline the decisions you need to make before you go out the door so all you need to do is *move*.

- **Set aside one drawer for clothes that you like moving in:** Keep a few pairs of leggings and sports bras, as well as some safe options for the days when sensory sensitivities make tight workout gear uncomfortable. Loose bottoms and loose T-shirts work well. You don't want hating the feeling of your clothes to be the reason you don't do your three-minute run. I've run in pajama tops before for this reason.

- **Nothing needs to match!** We all love days when we can wear our pretty workout sets with matching socks, perfect hair, and slicked eyebrows, but when you have a bad day of executive dysfunction or feel overstimulated, the last thing you need is to skip movement just because you don't feel like you look presentable. Style doesn't matter. Get used to wearing whatever is easiest to grab.

- **Do it for just one song:** Don't stare at a timer counting down the seconds. Cover that treadmill monitor and throw on a song that makes you *feel* something, that makes you feel like that future version of yourself. Build your tolerance over time. Some days you'll notice you can move for five songs, but sometimes just one is enough. All that matters is that you let the idea of "just one song" get you started.

- **If you miss a class because you were running late, remember that that's sometimes part of having ADHD:** Keep moving forward instead of getting trapped in a pit of anger at yourself. Quickly pick something else that's in front of you that you can do in that moment: a treadmill run, stretches, or push-ups.

- **If you're nervous about being at the gym, hop on the treadmill for an incline walk first thing:** As you walk, take a look around, create a map of the equipment in your head, and decide what you're going to do. Know that it's normal to feel unsure when you're in a new environment and that that feeling will pass with time as you get more comfortable.

- **Do the easiest thing:** We talk a lot about doing the hard thing first, but sometimes during really hard times, doing the easiest thing first will create the sense of accomplishment and build the momentum we need to boost our motivation. This tactic works especially well when the easy thing is also a novelty. After avoiding a gym workout for months, I decided to try something that I had never done before and made an appointment for soft-tissue therapy. Choosing the easiest thing at the time set off a domino effect of change (see page 17). The appointment lifted my energy enough for me to get myself to the gym after all that time, going to the gym led me to eating healthier, and eating healthier helped me sleep better at night.

Q: My schedule is already so packed, and I'm too tired at the end of the day to exercise. How can I make time for it?

A: Exercise will come last in your life if it's the last thing you get to in your day. If you try to exercise when your eyes are blurry and you're ready to collapse, you're not going to do it. You might find yourself thinking, *I don't want to, I can't be bothered,* or *It's 6:00 P.M. so the day is basically over. I might as well wait until tomorrow and do it properly!* These reasons may help us feel more comfortable in the moment, and that's fine now and again, or even for a season. You're human.

But when we let those thoughts dictate our actions in the long term, our confidence fades, our energy dims, and we lose respect for ourselves. We start to cement that age-old belief that we're just "naturally" unmotivated. A large part of making movement a habit is getting ourselves to think differently. To know that yes, someone who skipped movement is who we used to be, but now we are open and ready for change. Although it will be hard, it will get easier, and your effort will be worth it.

There's no special hack here, only some straight truth: Movement needs to be a priority. I know you can't put more on your plate, so it's time to consider taking something off it. Modern-day living can trap women with ADHD in a cycle of burnout. Saying yes to moving in some way—any way—is how you can break that cycle and bring more calm to your days.

This might mean you need to get creative with your schedule. You might try moving earlier in the day, before fatigue sets in. If you're struggling to find time for movement or feeling overwhelmed, online platforms are great because you don't need to think about getting out the door to make it on time to a class. There are so many options. Try out my Healthy Happy ADHD platform for ideas on adding some short bursts of low-impact movement to your day. Habit stacking (see page 27) will also help you incorporate movement into your everyday routine. And remember, you don't need to run a 5K or take a full forty-minute Pilates class to make it count.

# 5

## Add More Protein

*Instead of reducing food,*
*think about adding more food.*

Halfway through my running challenge, I started to notice a few changes for the better. I didn't have to coach myself as much to get out the door to run; the daily run felt like a priority in my life. I had more confidence in myself, because I was keeping my word to run every day. Another nice change was that the comfort eating I used to do had decreased. I naturally started craving more nutritious food, and the knock-on effect of eating more nutritious food was a more stable mood. I had fewer meltdowns and a clearer mind. Things were definitely looking up.

Despite the progress I had made, there was some room for improvement. I still felt heavy on my feet. I wanted to lose more of the weight I had gained in the past few years and feel agile, fit, and radiant. If I wanted to continue becoming the version of myself I saw in my daily visualization practice, it was time to put more focus on my nutrition.

It didn't take me long to figure out the missing piece in my nutritional puzzle. From working with thousands of women on their fitness journeys over the years, I had learned the transformative impact that protein can have on our minds and bodies. And I absolutely knew I wasn't getting enough of it at that time in my life. If I wanted to achieve the sort of mental and physical transformation I was hoping for, I was going to have to make an effort to add extra protein-rich foods to my plate. All I had to do was follow the same advice I had given so many others over the years to see the results first-hand.

## COUNT PROTEIN, NOT CALORIES

When it comes to healthy eating, I see many make the mistake of reducing calories to unhealthily low levels. I've seen fitness influencers demonize the avocado because its fat content is higher than that of other foods despite fat being the fuel of life for us women. I've seen others swap whole foods for fat-free alternatives and dubbing zero-calorie foods and sauces their heroes. I used to do this too. When I think about one of those zero-calorie sauces now, I gag. It's no wonder I had gut health issues with all those strange ingredients going into my body multiple times a day.

We can argue about the virtues of "calories in, calories out" all day long, but I believe there is a lot more to food than the number of calories we take in. **What we eat directly impacts our brain chemistry, blood sugar level, gut health, and inflammation level, all of which play a part in our energy level and mood (which ADHD women tend to struggle with).** Many foods contain compounds that boost brain health—for example, celery, beets, and blueberries. In fact, there isn't one part of the body that food *doesn't* impact. The calorie count of a meal doesn't represent its full power to transform not only how we look, but how we *feel*.

You don't need to lose your health, your joy, or your life to eat healthy. You don't need to lose your health in the pursuit of losing weight. You don't need to feel so hungry that it affects your mood and relationships. You don't need to be so stressed about calories that it affects your hormones and relationship with food. Nor do you need to feel so exhausted that it affects your outlook on life. It's crucial that you set up habits that help you live in harmony with yourself and the world around you, especially when it comes to something you need to do every day.

**When I took a closer look at my nutrition, I wanted to think more about what I could add to my plate instead of**

**focusing on what I should cut out.** I knew I wouldn't stick with a restrictive calorie-based diet because it wouldn't be enjoyable seven days a week. Sure, you can count calories and track every morsel of food you eat, but does that sound like a solid, healthy, and happy *lifetime* plan? For me, the answer was no. I had no desire to start tracking every morsel of food I ate on a fitness app. I didn't want to cut out all the foods that I love, like my favorite ice cream. Not to mention that counting calories takes a lot of executive function. It requires extra thinking, organizing, and planning. And when calorie counting doesn't go according to plan, it can bring up feelings of failure.

When it came to my relationship with food, focusing on adding instead of subtracting would also put me in a much healthier frame of mind and would help me enjoy my favorite foods without guilt or shame. Sometimes we just need that chocolate doughnut for the dopamine hit. Forcing ourselves to track calories on some app and justify what we want to eat isn't what we need when we're already tapped out.

I want you to thrive, not just survive, as a woman with ADHD. **When we focus on adding foods that help us feel our best, we can learn to trust our bodies to tell us what they need and honor those needs.**

## WHY PROTEIN MATTERS

When I asked myself what I could *add* to my diet to achieve my goals, my answer was protein—and for good reason. Protein is essential for our health and well-being, and vital for healthy, sustainable body transformation, especially if you have ADHD. This key nutrient can bolster brain health and help us avoid mood dips, hormonal issues, and more.

### Protein Supports Our ADHD Brains

Our brains often have low levels of important feel-good neu-rotransmitters such as dopamine and norepinephrine. This regularly leaves us feeling tired, moody, and unmotivated, and our brains itchy for stimulation. Protein-rich foods like turkey, eggs, legumes, beans, and beef are full of the amino acids that help produce these neurotransmitters. And they do so without the crash that happens after eating a lot of our go-to dopamine-spiking comfort foods, like pizza or cookies.

Some studies even suggest that protein and its ability to curb these crashes could be helpful with our more frustrating ADHD symptoms. For example, researchers found that in-corporating protein into our diets can help keep our blood sugar level from rising too much, which might lessen the se-verity of ADHD symptoms in adults.

Protein can also support our mental health. Multiple studies have shown that people with ADHD are at an increased risk of experiencing depression. A 2020 paper found that people who ate more protein generally had fewer depressive symptoms. More specifically, when people ate about one gram of protein per kilogram of body weight a day, their risk of depressive symptoms fell.

## Protein Keeps Us Satiated and Energized

Eating more protein can be a hard habit to start if you've been taught not to eat too much. But trust me: If you do this, you'll find yourself much fuller after meals and experience fewer cravings. You'll still enjoy chocolate, but you'll feel less compelled to eat six bars at once when you indulge.

Protein keeps you feeling full because it takes longer to digest than carbs and fats. This slower digestion also helps stabilize your blood sugar level, preventing rapid spikes and crashes that can lead to increased hunger and cravings. Protein-rich foods trigger the release of satiety hormones, hormones that send a message to the brain that you're full and satisfied.

Without enough protein intake, you might feel weak and have less energy and motivation. This, in turn, leaves us more likely to reach for less nutritious foods or engage in *any* behavior that brings change.

Remember: More protein→Fewer cravings→Better moods, more energy

## Protein Supports Body Recomposition

If you want to manage your weight or look leaner, what you're looking to do is undergo body recomposition. With body recomposition, you reduce your body fat while maintaining or increasing muscle. This will give you that lean look, because muscle takes up less space than the equivalent weight of fat.

Incorporating more protein will support muscle maintenance and new muscle growth. Protein is the building block for your muscles. When you exercise, the stress on your muscles causes tiny tears. Protein helps repair these tears, making your muscles stronger over time. It also helps replenish energy stores and supports overall recovery.

Years ago, when I started out as a health-and-fitness coach, new clients who heard the words "more protein" would often tell me they didn't want to get all big and muscular, *like those guys*. Before you yell, "*I don't want to look bulky*," let me say this: There is no scenario where you wake up one morning and find that you've turned into a massive bodybuilder.

I promise, those guys did not get all big and muscular by accident. Most people can only gain between one-half and two pounds of muscle per month. Building bulky muscles demands a *lot* more effort than upping your protein intake. Creating a physique like that also requires you to up your caloric intake and follow a very specific resistance-training program. Sure, some people's genetics prime them to gain muscle faster than others, but remember that your genetics only loads the gun. It's your lifestyle choices and what you do daily that pulls the trigger to get results—or a lack of results.

The process of building bulky muscles is even more challenging if you're a woman. Women have less testosterone, a hormone that plays a big role in muscle growth. As a result, we aren't as likely to experience the same bulky results that men get when following similar diets and workout routines.

Protein alone does *not* make you bulky. If anything, upping your protein intake will help you sculpt your body. Having more muscle increases your metabolism, which means you'll use more energy while resting than the person with less muscle does. I can confirm that protein is a game changer based on my firsthand experience. I was working out nonstop throughout my hundred-day running challenge. There wasn't much change in my body composition until I became mindful of my protein intake.

## Protein Supports Metabolic Health

When you eat food, your body breaks it down into sugar, which enters the bloodstream. Your pancreas releases the hormone insulin to transport the sugar from the blood into the cells, and the cells in your body convert this sugar into energy. The liver stores any extra sugar for later, lowering your blood sugar and insulin levels. When there is too much sugar in the bloodstream, the pancreas pumps out more insulin. If this abnormal state continues over the long term, your body stops responding to insulin and you eventually become insulin resistant. Your diet is not the only thing that can cause this—chronic stress and trauma also contribute to insulin resistance. We will get into these other factors more later in the book, but in this chapter we will primarily be focusing on diet.

**Insulin resistance occurs when your body has trouble using insulin properly, which can cause a bunch of health problems, including type 2 diabetes.** Insulin resistance is also often linked to obesity and higher levels of visceral fat around the midsection, which can raise your chances of having heart issues. An elevated insulin level can prompt the ovaries to produce excessive testosterone, which interferes with normal ovulation. In fact, there is a strong link between insulin resistance and polycystic ovary syndrome (PCOS), which can lead to irregular periods, ovarian cysts, acne, and excess facial and body hair growth. More than half of women with PCOS will be diagnosed with type 2 diabetes by age forty.

Incorporating protein into your meals, particularly during the first and last meals of the day, can be a helpful strategy for managing blood sugar levels and potentially reducing the risk of insulin resistance. Protein has a lesser impact on blood sugar compared to carbohydrates, and eating protein and fats alongside carbs can slow their digestion and help stabilize blood sugar so the pancreas doesn't have to produce as much insulin. This is why you experience stable energy levels and fewer cravings when you have a few eggs with your bagel instead of eating a bagel on its own. The same happens when you have lentils with rice instead of rice alone.

## TIPS FOR BLOOD SUGAR BALANCE

Protein isn't the only way to keep your blood sugar level in check. Here are some other strategies for keeping it balanced:

- Choose somewhat underripe produce like slightly green bananas, which have less of an effect on blood sugar than ripened produce.
- Eat foods in their whole-food forms. This means leaving skin on veggies like potatoes. The fiber in the skin helps slow digestion, moderating the sugar spike.
- If juicing, use low-sugar veggies and fruits such as celery and cucumber.
- Add veggies, such as carrots, broccoli, cauliflower, peppers, mushrooms, turnips, and parsnips, to your meals. When eating out, opt for a starter of vegetables.
- When you can, swap low-fiber carbs such as white rice for high-fiber carbs such as quinoa.
- Aim for balanced meals and snacks with good sources of protein and fats and high-fiber carbohydrates.

- Check ingredients labels for added sugars. Flavored yogurts are a big culprit.

- Practice regular movement to help your body use glucose more effectively, which can prevent blood sugar spikes. Going for a quick walk or doing some squats after a meal makes your body use sugar for energy instead of letting it build up in the blood.

- Build your muscles. When there's less muscle tissue, the body's ability to use glucose decreases. Plus, lower muscle mass often correlates with higher body fat percentage. Excess body fat, especially visceral fat around organs, releases inflammatory substances, changes your hormone levels, and reduces insulin sensitivity in muscle cells.

- Be mindful of stress. When you're stressed, your body releases cortisol and adrenaline (also known as epinephrine), hormones that tell the liver to release stored sugar that your body might not need into the bloodstream. If you then eat sugary foods to try to feel relief and comfort, your blood sugar can spike even more. Stress becomes a double whammy, raising your blood sugar and leading you to sugary comfort foods that make it spike even higher.

## HOW MUCH PROTEIN?

For most of our lives, we have been led to believe that we need less protein than most of us actually do. In fact, research shows the average moderately active person may need about 41 to 50 percent more protein than we were previously told was necessary.

If we go by official government regulations and recommendations, we're often just getting enough to survive. But what if we want to thrive? Recommended dietary allowance (RDA) numbers don't account for optimal health and longevity. **I recommend eating around 1.5 to 2 grams of protein per kilogram of body weight per day** to feel better both mentally and physically.

You don't have to make extra meals to get what you need. Simply adding an extra protein source to the meal you're already eating or increasing the amount of a protein-rich food on your plate will work. First, you'll need to know how much protein you need. I'll give you three options for calculating the amount of protein. Start with one, and if it feels like too much to eat, shift to another method if you want to. You won't feel restricted to one number, and regardless of which option you pick, you will feel at ease knowing you are eating more protein than before.

## Option One: 2 Grams

What's your body weight in kilograms? _____

Multiply that number by two. _____

Easy peasy.

If your weight is 50 kilograms, aim to eat 100 grams of protein per day.

If your weight is 75 kilograms, aim to eat 150 grams of protein per day.

If your weight is 100 kilograms, aim to eat 200 grams of protein per day.

## Option Two: 1.5 Grams

What's your body weight in kilograms? _____

Multiply that number by 1.5. _____

Easy peasy.

If your weight is 50 kilograms, aim to eat 75 grams of protein per day.

If your weight is 75 kilograms, aim to eat about 110 grams of protein per day.

If your weight is 100 kilograms, aim to eat 150 grams of protein per day.

## Option Three: Double Your Protein

If calculating a specific amount feels like too much for you right now or if you don't want to work with a specific number, the hack for eating more protein can truly be as simple as doubling the amount of protein that you're already eating. For example, when you're ordering a turkey sandwich, ask for extra turkey. If you usually eat two eggs with toast, aim to eat four.

With all three options, I emphasize *aiming* to hit these guidelines. I want to stress how important it is that you take the amounts given above as approximations. They aren't something to seek perfection on or be obsessed with. **Think of these numbers as rough benchmarks—you don't need to count every morsel of food or treat every meal like a math equation. The point of this pillar is to simply add more protein to whatever you're already eating.** There will be times when you will have more protein than these amounts, maybe because you are undergoing an intense period of athletic training. There will also be times when you eat less because life happens . . . well, specifically, *life with ADHD* happens.

You're not going to get every gram of protein every single day, but when you aim for the number you calculated on page 146, I guarantee you'll be eating more of it than you used to.

Shooting for this ballpark number might even become second nature.


## Build Your Protein Blocks

Once you have your protein number, it's helpful to figure out which high-protein foods you like and get a rough understanding of how much of each to eat. To keep things simple, I think of my high-protein foods as 30-gram "blocks."

I like using 30 grams as a guideline because it roughly corresponds to the serving sizes of common high-protein foods, so the amount of food for each block is easy to remember. Thirty grams of protein[*] looks like:

- One chicken breast

- Four eggs

- One can of tuna

- A serving of high-quality protein powder

This adds up to approximately 120 grams of protein for the day.

On top of these blocks, you can get more protein through-

[*] The protein quantity may depend on the quality of the food and the country you are in.

out the day by adding some nuts and nut butters, seeds, and legumes to meals and snacks (see "Easy Protein Ideas" on page 150 for more details).

If you don't eat foods from animals, here's what 30 grams of protein looks like in plant-based options. A measuring cup is a must-have until you can eyeball the measurements.

- 1½ cups tofu

- 1½ cups lentils

- 1 cup cashew nuts

- 1 cup chia seeds

- ¾ cup chickpeas

- 2 cups black beans

It's important to note that meat and eggs are considered complete protein sources because they provide all the essential amino acids that the body needs for protein synthesis and various other physiological functions. Some plant-based sources have low levels of certain essential amino acids. Mixing various plant proteins and eating a diverse range of plant-based foods throughout the day is crucial so you get adequate amounts of all the essential amino acids you need. For example, if you want to eat a chickpea curry, you can get all the essential amino acids by adding peas to the curry and eating it with quinoa.

## Easy Protein Ideas

- **Add legumes:** Throw a handful of peas or beans into meals such as curries and stir-fries for an easy extra boost of protein alongside the meat you're cooking.

- **Add nuts and seeds:** Add a dash of nuts or seeds to oatmeal, salads, smoothies, and stir-fries and buy seeded breads and crackers instead of plain ones.

- **Upgrade your toast:** Toast is a great blank canvas for protein-rich toppings. Nut butters and cottage cheese are some of the easiest options. Try smoked salmon or hummus topped with tomato or cucumber for a more satisfying snack.

- **Upgrade your base:** Quinoa is a great alternative to rice because it's packed with extra nutrients. Unlike rice, which primarily provides just carbohydrates, quinoa is a complete protein, meaning it contains all nine essential amino acids. It also provides fiber, vitamins, and minerals such as magnesium, iron, and zinc.

- **Turkey or chicken slices:** Roll up slices of deli turkey or chicken breast for a quick and easy protein-packed snack on the go. Add some cheese, nuts, and an apple or dip the roll-ups in hummus for extra satiety and flavor.

**Q:** I get why protein is important, but when I'm looking for a snack, I'm more likely to turn to my favorite carb-heavy foods. What are my options?

**A:** I notice when I am doubling my protein and eating protein-rich meals, my energy level is more stable and I'm not reaching for carb-heavy snacks so much between meals. If you still find yourself snacking a lot between meals, it could be a sign that you need to eat bigger meals or increase the amount of protein and fiber that you're already eating.

That said, sometimes you just want a snack. While you're starting to adopt new, healthy eating habits, a good rule of thumb is just to add some protein to the snack you're craving. If you want a bagel, spread some almond butter on it. If you're eating crackers, top them with a few slices of turkey.

Remember, we are focusing on *adding* rather than restricting. Food is fuel, but food is also fun. There's no planet I live on where I say no to birthday cake. I *could* add some protein so I don't feel slumped and sleepy after the birthday cake, but I'm not obsessing over eating something I want to eat. The more you practice this way of eating, the more you'll notice yourself intuitively adding foods to your plate just because they're good for you instead of taking things away from your plate because they're over your calorie count for the day.

# 6

## Simplify Your Relationship with Food

*Food has power, and what we eat*
*affects how we feel.*

When I think back to the successful health and life-style changes I've made in the past, they've had one thing in common: I was eating well.

When I eat well, I have more energy for life. And when I have more energy for life, I can tackle the small things that can be easy to neglect. I'm able to wash the dishes instead of leaving them in a pile for days. I have clean clothes fresh out of the laundry. I don't skip my skin-care routine at night. I actually feel like chopping the overripe bananas and putting them in the freezer instead of letting them rot and gather fruit flies. Eventually, these small things add up to improve my overall quality of life. It means that I don't have to live in a house where food is rotting, dishes are piling up, and clean socks are hard to find.

This might be common sense to you, but the way we feed

our bodies directly correlates to how we feel and function. This can be either good or bad news, depending on your current eating habits. If you want to become healthy and happy, you'll want to make sure you're getting the nutrients that help you feel that way. And because you have ADHD, you'll want to do this without relying on discipline, adding to your already overflowing mental load, or following any rules around food.

I discovered that making healthy eating doable for me came down to these four habits: being curious about what I ate and why I ate it, making my meals as easy as possible, building meals around protein, and eating the same meals on repeat to avoid decision fatigue. We'll cover how each of these habits helps us tackle the obstacles that make eating nutritious foods feel impossible.

## GET CURIOUS ABOUT YOUR EATING PATTERNS

After I began paying attention to my protein intake and noticing how it made me feel stronger and more energized, I became curious about how different types and combinations of foods affected my energy and mood. I liked getting this instant feedback from my body. I noticed how exhausted I felt after having a big plate of pasta at lunch.

Following this curiosity helped me realize that we eat for

many reasons, not just hunger. This is especially true if you have ADHD. Your brain's natural tendencies impact how you fuel your body—and that can make healthy eating especially difficult.

As someone with ADHD, there's a strong chance that you often reach for food when you're understimulated or bored. This is one of the key reasons many women with ADHD struggle with their relationship with food. When there isn't enough sensory input from the world around you, you might have trouble staying engaged with whatever you're doing at that moment. You might start to feel restless and look for immediate stimulation. In many instances, this happens without you being consciously aware of it or thinking about it. It's like an automatic reflex—your brain is underaroused and bored, and it wants a party. Resisting the urge to find stimulation can feel like you're fighting against yourself. Because food provides the stimulation that our brain craves, we might find ourselves peeking in our kitchen cupboards even if we just ate breakfast, simply because we want something interesting to do.

In addition to stimulation, food often brings comfort when we're feeling stressed, helping to take the edge off. While occasionally turning to a favorite dish or snack after a bad day isn't anything to worry about, it's a hard habit to break if you fall back on it in the long term. When we're overwhelmed, we might not be able to curb our impulse to comfort eat. To make matters worse, comfort eating might make us feel out of control or ashamed that we're not taking care of ourselves. This adds fuel to the emotional fire—because comfort eating makes us feel bad about ourselves, we might wind up doing more of it to deal with those uncomfortable emotions.

## EATING FOR STIMULATION ISN'T BINGE EATING

Like many people with ADHD, I tend to snack a lot for stimulation. I call this tendency ADHD dopamine snacking. You could call it boredom eating, and you could consider it comfort eating to an extent. What it isn't, though, is binge eating.

In one study, women with ADHD were 3.6 times more likely to have an eating disorder than those without ADHD. The most common eating disorder of those women was binge eating disorder. Binge eating is when you eat a large amount of food in a short window of time (an hour or two). Having an extra bowl of ice cream when you're stressed doesn't mean you're experiencing disordered eating, but you might be if you secretly binge over a period of months; feel out of control during these episodes; and feel disgust, shame, and guilt afterward. Binge eating is often a response to emotional pain and could be a sign that you're holding trauma in your body.

Back in my late teens and early twenties, before I started my health-and-fitness career, I experienced a few episodes of disordered eating. In hindsight, I can see that I had the obvious signs of an eating disorder, and if I had asked for help back then, I might have been diagnosed with one. I once bought a whole cake, ate half of it, and threw it in the garbage bin to hide the evidence, only to go back to the bin to eat more the next morning. I felt embarrassed and on edge when eating in front of people, and for a long time I was hypervigilant about people watching me eat (spoiler alert: they weren't). If I had been diagnosed with ADHD at a young age, I might have used medication in a destructive way to curb my appetite because of the headspace I was in at the time. If you think you are dealing with an eating disorder, please know that help is available. If possible, seek out a healthcare professional who has experience in treating eating disorders and is also ADHD informed so you can feel as heard and understood as possible.

## Curiosity Will Be Your Guide

Eating for stimulation or comfort isn't always a big deal, but it can become a problem if you mindlessly eat when you're not hungry and when the food you reach for affects you negatively. For instance, maybe you get uncomfortably bloated every night as a result of the foods you're eating. I find that many women who are trying to get healthier or fitter think they need to cut out all their favorite foods, swapping in low-calorie options or stopping snacking altogether, but that's not the case. Instead of fighting the urge to snack for stimulation, create space for it. When you allow and create space for something, you'll be less likely to obsess over it or feel like you're missing out.

---

*When you allow and create space for something, you'll be less likely to obsess over it or feel like you're missing out.*

---

The key again is to turn to your curiosity. This time, consider the way you eat. What do you feel in your body when you're about to reach for a comfort snack? Does this happen at a certain time of day or when you're trying to do a certain task? **The answers to these questions help us become more aware of our patterns, and when we're armed with this knowledge, it becomes easier to figure out the best way to give your body what it needs.**

Building this self-awareness isn't easy at first, and you won't always remember to do it or have the energy to think twice when confronting a craving. **Instead of fighting the craving and denying the feeling, allow it to come up and ask yourself, *Am I hungry?***

If the answer is yes, then you need to eat! If you've already eaten a meal and are still hungry, make sure you're using the guidance given in the last chapter to increase your protein intake, which will help keep you full.

Not hungry? Try putting what you're feeling into words:

- *I'm not hungry, I'm bored.*

- *I'm not hungry, I feel stressed.*

- *I'm not hungry, I want chocolate.*

Once you're able to put your finger on what your body really wants, you'll often be able to nourish it in a more meaningful way. For example, sometimes when I need stimulation to focus on a boring task, I pour myself a glass of icy sparkling water with half a lemon squeezed into it. The sharpness of the sparkling water and the zest of the lemon just *do something* to my brain, giving me the kick I need to stay on task. Other times, I want a snack to tide me over until dinner or before a session at the gym. In that case, I try to find something that won't spike my blood sugar or give me an energy crash. (There are some simple snack ideas on page 170.) If I really just want chocolate, I'll try to eat it with some nuts to help balance my blood sugar and avoid a sugar high and crash. I keep a clear glass jar of nuts on my countertop just for moments like this (again, if it's in sight, it's in mind).

You might also eat something because it's part of something fun. Food is associated with lots of positive experiences in our lives. We eat with friends and family to celebrate and to connect. We eat when we're enjoying our favorite activities. The cinema is one of my favorite places in the world. I love sitting in front of the big screen in a cool, dark room where all I can hear is the movie and I'm able to happily ignore my phone and the outside world. My go-to movie snack is ice cream (one scoop of cookie dough and one scoop of peanut butter in a cup, please), popcorn, and hot tea. I put popcorn on top of the ice cream as I'm eating it, and I'm as happy as can be with this sensory experience. I look forward to the snacks as much as the movie.

It's possible to be healthy without feeling shame for the moments when we eat for escapism and fun. **What you feel about the food you eat is as important as the food itself!** Feeling guilt or shame for eating something can dampen the release of those happy hormones and even trigger the release of stress hormones such as cortisol. Emotions associated with guilt or shame can interfere with the brain's reward system, potentially impacting mood and overall well-being.

How you interact with food is something to notice in your life, not a reason to beat yourself up for enjoying an ice cream at the cinema. You don't need to shame yourself for moments of peace and joy or for not always having the healthiest option on hand. Sometimes the stress of trying to eat perfectly hurts you more than the food you're trying to avoid or simply doing the best you can from moment to moment.

---

*You don't need to shame yourself for moments of peace and joy or for not always having the healthiest option on hand.*

---

## THE SENSORY SNACK BOWL

When we refer to "junk food," we're typically talking about ultra-processed foods. Think things like potato chips or candy. A small serving of these sorts of foods is rarely satisfying, leaving you reaching for more and leading to overconsumption. Most of us are all too familiar with the bloated, sluggish, and even unwell feeling that follows finishing off a family-size bag of potato chips.

You might have heard people saying it's the sugar in these foods that's addictive. Or maybe it's the salt. Or the fat. But the fact of the matter is that there's not just one element to blame. It's the combination of sugar, salt, fat, texture, and shape that hooks you.

These foods are strategically designed to be convenient, highly palatable, and addictive. Food scientists and product creators spend hours and millions of dollars on creating the perfect blend of sweetness and richness to trigger your brain's pleasure centers, leaving you craving more and buying more. It's this intentional blending that creates the addictive feeling, the feeling of "I can't stop"—the makers of Pringles even said it themselves in an advertising slogan: "Once you pop, you can't stop!"—driving you to either eat way more than you intended or waste loads of energy trying to harness enough willpower to resist the craving.

So what are we supposed to do about our junk food cravings? Opting for a healthy treat over an unhealthy one seems like a simple enough option, but it can be difficult at times. For starters, the healthier option might not taste as good. No, really. Some research suggests artificial sweeteners found in our favorite ultra-processed treats can dull our taste buds over time, reducing sensitivity to the flavors of whole foods and making the natural flavors less satisfying in comparison. Simply taking some time away from these foods could restore the sensitivity in your taste buds, but as I just said, resisting cravings takes willpower. And that can be difficult to muster after a tough day when we're already exhausted and want to just numb out. Another suggestion that people often throw out there is to practice moderation. But what does that even mean? Moderation looks different to every individual.

**For me, only one solution has really done the trick: the Sensory Snack Bowl.**

The Sensory Snack Bowl is what I call a snack that offers a

mix of different textures and tastes: sweet, salty, savory, crunchy, cold, hot, all at once. I don't want to restrict myself or cut out certain foods that I enjoy, but I also don't want to eat massive portions of ultra-processed foods and struggle with poor digestion and low energy. So I snack smarter.

I simply go for what I'm craving and add in some contrasting tastes and textures. For instance, one of my favorite Sensory Snack Bowls starts with a scoop of good quality ice cream or frozen yogurt, topped with salty popcorn. I'll add some seeds and nuts to the bowl for crunch, and because they also give me some fats, fiber, and protein, which help reduce the sugar spike from the ice cream and prevent an energy crash. Some of my Sensory Snack Bowls include foods that I can fidget with, which can help with self-soothing. Think grapes, for example. If you're like me, you peel off the skin first. A chocolate bar with a biscuit in the middle, which you might eat by nibbling the outside of the bar first, also helps me keep my hands busy.

Unlike potato chips, which are easy to mindlessly eat in excessive quantities because all the chips taste the same, the complex sensory experience from the Sensory Snack Bowl's diverse tastes and textures activates multiple sensory pathways simultaneously, leading to heightened neural activity and stimulation in the brain and promoting relaxation. It also keeps you in the present. Noticing the contrasts and sensations from the Sensory Snack Bowl can help you feel calm and grounded.

If you're sensitive to certain textures or tastes, experiencing different sensations all at once may be overwhelming or dysregulating. When I used to struggle with premenstrual dysphoric disorder (PMDD), there were times of the month when I couldn't handle the sound of crunching because my sensory processing was much more sensitive. Choosing foods that suit you and being aware of how certain foods affect you will help you better connect with what feels good.

## MEET THE ADHD EASY MEAL

When it comes to cooking, it's all about convenience.

When there are too many steps involved with cooking a meal, it's just way easier to reach for takeout. If there are too many rules about what I'm "supposed" to eat, I get stuck in analysis paralysis.

My idea of convenience is not prepping all my meals and portioning them into Tupperware containers on Sunday night. To be honest, I leave most of the food uneaten because I have a fear of food poisoning, and I don't like the texture of some foods after they've been sitting awhile in the fridge. I would rather throw together something easy and fast.

This is where ADHD Easy Meals come in. This is the name I coined to describe simple, fuss-free ways of eating that helped me feed myself without the stress, overwhelm, and analysis paralysis. An ADHD Easy Meal checks off these boxes:

- It's fast

- It requires little prep or cleanup

- It's nutritious

- It's easy to modify

You don't need a hundred-recipe cookbook to come up with ideas for your ADHD Easy Meals. Flipping through a book, choosing a recipe, checking to see if you have the ingredients, finding those ingredients if you don't, and following fifteen step-by-step instructions isn't always easy for my brain to get on board with. Now and again? Sure! But for everyday life, you just need a few simple options that you can turn to time and again. **ADHD Easy Meals are about dropping the rules and finding efficiency however you can.** I know cooking traditionally involves multiple steps: heat the oil, add some garlic, wait a minute until the garlic's browned, then add the tomato paste and pepper, wait for two more minutes, then add the mushrooms, let them brown. . . . I'd rather throw everything in a pan at the same time and be done, thank you. Although the traditional way may taste better, my way tastes just as good to me because I didn't waste time thinking about all the steps.

## Build Your Plate

You can make an ADHD Easy Meal out of anything once you know how to build your plate. **Building your plate is as simple as asking yourself these two questions:** *What protein do I have on hand?* **and** *What can I add to make that a meal?* This lets you skip the decisions that often make cooking so hard and focus on the ones that actually help you eat better. You don't need to worry about running to the store if you don't have an ingredient.

This strategy, as with many in the book, has a lot of built-in flexibility. It works whether I want something very specific or I just need to eat something right now. It still works if you get tired of one dish out of the blue and want something new. It doesn't ask you to follow any rules about what foods should go together and when they should be eaten. Sometimes, you want a bowl of oatmeal for dinner, and that's okay.

Depending on where in the world you're located and your personal preferences, the foods that work best for you may look different. Here's an example of some foods I use to build my plate (there are many more you can add):

## Step 1: Pick a High-Protein Food

Chicken breast or thighs

Turkey breast or thighs

Lean cut of beef

Turkey bacon or rashers

Whitefish

Salmon

Sardines

Eggs

Protein powder

Legumes such as lentils, chickpeas, and black beans

Tofu

## Step 2: Add a Fat

Avocado

Nuts and nut butters (for instance, almonds, cashews,
    walnuts, Brazil nuts, hazelnuts)**

Chia seeds

Ground flaxseeds

Eggs*

Olives or olive oil

Coconut milk or oil

Full-fat Greek yogurt

Salmon* (a good omega-3 fat source)

Sardines* (a good omega-3 fat source)

*Fatty fish and eggs are also rich in healthy fats and can count as both a protein and a fat source.

**Nuts are also rich in protein.

## Step 3: Add a Carb

Quinoa

Brown rice

Oats

Potato (with the skin)

Corn tortillas

Pita or sourdough bread

Legumes such as lentils, chickpeas, and black beans*

Root vegetables such as carrots, and squash (with the skin)

Fruits such as bananas, berries, apples, and oranges

*Legumes contain complex carbohydrates and can count as both a protein and a carb source.

## Step 4: Add Color with Vegetables and Fruits

Peppers

Mushrooms

Carrots

Broccoli

Peas

Apples

Pears

Pineapple

Cherries

Blueberries

## Step 5: Pick Your Flavors

Herbs (such as basil, oregano, rosemary, parsley)

Spices (such as black pepper, garam masala, curry powder, turmeric, paprika, Ceylon cinnamon)

Here are some examples of how I use these steps to create ADHD Easy Meals:

**The ADHD Easy Meal:** high-protein breakfast shake
**What's my protein?** Protein powder
**What else can I add?**

- Fat: almond butter
- Carb: banana
- Vegetable or fruit: berries
- Flavor: cinnamon

**The ADHD Easy Meal:** high-protein breakfast oatmeal
**What's my protein?** Protein powder

**What else can I add?**

- Fat: chia seeds
- Carb: oats
- Vegetable or fruit: blueberries
- Flavor: cinnamon

**The ADHD Easy Meal:** Burrito bowl

**What's my protein?** Ground beef

**What else can I add?**

- Fat: smashed avocado
- Carb: rice
- Vegetable or fruit: peppers, tomatoes, lettuce
- Flavor: paprika

**The ADHD Easy Meal:** Egg tacos

**What's my protein?** Eggs

**What else can I add?**

- Fat: avocado
- Carb: corn tortillas
- Vegetable or fruit: peppers
- Flavor: hot sauce

**The ADHD Easy Meal:** Chicken curry

**What's my protein?** Chicken

**What else can I add?**

- Fat: coconut milk
- Carb: quinoa

- Vegetable or fruit: green beans, mushrooms
- Flavor: curry powder, garam masala, paprika

**The ADHD Easy Meal:** My "I forgot to eat" snack plate
**What's my protein?** Smoked salmon
**What else can I add?**

- Fat: hummus
- Carb: seeded crackers
- Vegetable or fruit: cucumber, tomato
- Flavor: pickles

Over time, you'll get so used to making meals this way that you'll be able to throw them together with your eyes closed, freeing up your brain space for something else.

## Easy Snack Ideas That Won't Give You an Energy Crash

Need a quick snack to hold you over? You can build energy-sustaining snacks in the same way that you build your plate to create a meal by starting with a protein and then adding your fat, carb, fruit or vegetable, and flavor. Depending on how much time and energy you have, you can skip some of these components as long as you have a good source of protein.

The following combinations are easy, delicious, and nutritious:

- Almond butter + cinnamon + banana on sourdough bread

- Apple slices + almond butter + sea salt

- Banana + a handful of nuts + a square of dark chocolate

- Greek yogurt + protein powder + berries

- Leftover roasted chicken + tomato + crackers

- Hummus + chicken + pita

## EAT MORE PLANTS

You might have grown up hearing that you need to eat five servings of fruits and vegetables a day for optimal health. Research has found it's not just the number of plants that matters, but the variety. It's now thought that consuming about thirty different plants a week is just as important as eating five servings of them a day.

Researchers at the American Gut Project found that people who ate more than thirty different plant foods each week had a more diverse gut microbiome than those who ate ten or fewer. They also had more gut bacteria that produce short-chain fatty acids during the fermentation of dietary fiber, which provide energy to colon cells, reduce inflammation, support gut health, and help regulate metabolism.

A healthy and diverse gut microbiome is important because the gut and brain are connected through a complex communication network known as the gut-brain axis. It plays a crucial role in regulating neurotransmitter production, immune function, and inflammation levels—all of which can influence brain function and mental health. Imbalances in the gut microbiome have been linked to attention issues, mood disturbances, and behavioral problems. Research in the field of microbiome science and neurology is ongoing, but there is a growing body of evidence supporting these associations.

This doesn't mean you have to get thirty full servings of veggies a week (I'd find that extremely hard). The good news is that all plants count, even in small quantities. Nuts, seeds, even a pinch of an herb or spice can go toward meeting your total. It can be as easy as adding paprika, oregano, or black pepper to your dinner; sprinkling cinnamon on your snacks; putting some slices of lemon, ginger, and cucumber in your sparkling water; and drinking a cup of herbal tea made from rose, spearmint, or chamomile. Keeping a range of herbs, spices, and teas in your cupboards can make it easy to increase the diversity of the plants you get in a week. Once a month, I fill up a jar with a mixture of seeds (chia, flax, pumpkin) and another with a mixture of nuts (walnuts, almonds, cashews, pistachios). Adding small amounts of these nuts and seeds to my yogurt along with a sprinkle of cinnamon and a handful of blueberries and strawberries, and pairing it with a cup of spearmint tea is already giving me eleven plants in one snack. See how easy it can be?

## Grocery Shopping Hacks

The ADHD Easy Meal is even easier when you keep your cupboards and freezer stocked with the foods that you use the most. Having what you need makes your life in the kitchen easy. And when your life in the kitchen is easy, fueling your body becomes easy.

I'm not sure exactly what you like to eat on a weekly basis, so I can't tell you exactly what to have on hand at all times. But here are the items that I keep on hand to minimize prep work and cleanup as much as I can:

- **Frozen or prechopped veggies and fruits:** The fewer things you have to slice, dice, and chop, the better. My favorite prechopped veggies to have on hand are peppers and onions. In my freezer, I keep garden peas to throw in all types of dishes, from curries to stews to stir-fries, and lots of blueberries for my protein shakes. Avoid canned fruits and veggies, because the skins are often removed before canning and they may contain added sugar or salt.

- **Condiments, sauces, and staple ingredients with a long shelf life:** Think coconut milk, canned chopped tomatoes or tomato puree, a jar of mustard, and a bottle of hot sauce.

- **Jars of minced garlic and minced ginger:** Never chop these yourself again!

- **Easy sources of protein:** In my kitchen, you'll find a large container of protein powder. When I want to throw together a quick but filling meal, it's a lifesaver to toss a serving into a bowl of Greek yogurt or oats or blend it with a shake. If I have time, I'll pop a whole chicken into the oven on a Monday so I have cooked meat for the next couple of days. I can make chicken sandwiches, chicken omelets, chicken fajitas, chicken curry, and many other dishes without too much thought because it's already cooked.

- **Herbs and spices:** Herbs and spices do more than add flavor. If you're hyperfixating on a specific flavor, you can use herbs and spices to turn an ADHD Easy Meal into something you're truly excited to eat.

- **Canned beans and microwavable pouches of rice, quinoa, and lentils:** Using these options is so much easier than cooking them from scratch.

If you're anything like me, walking through a busy supermarket can feel overstimulating and exhausting. The endless choices, the noise, people bumping into each other, the long lines, the bright lights, and the constant distractions can easily throw me off track, leaving me frazzled. Plus, I make so many more unhealthy impulse buys in supermarkets. I take these two approaches to grocery shopping to combat this:

1. I like to integrate food shopping into my routine as mentioned in chapter 1, when I talked about stacking habits. Swinging by the butcher after grabbing my morning coffee during my morning dog walk reduces decision fatigue and makes groceries something that I don't have to find extra energy to get. I also know where to find exactly what I need without the distractions, and I feel more a part of my local community when I see familiar faces in local stores, which is a great mental health bonus.

2. I regularly use online shopping apps and subscriptions. I live in a city, so it's easy to order groceries and have them delivered within thirty minutes or to set up a subscription to a store or farm to deliver the same foods each week at a set price. This helps me get the exact foods I need without the challenges of navigating a supermarket or setting aside time to visit one each week.

These strategies have higher up-front costs, but they've actually saved me money in the long run because I'm not impulse buying in the store. Online, you can stick to your shopping list more effectively and avoid distractions that often lead to overspending in physical stores. Many online platforms also offer discounts, subscription benefits, and bulk-buying options that can help you stick to your budget.

## Low-Effort Cooking Styles

Cooking doesn't mean you need to have four pots simmering on the stove. I cook that way at times, of course, but to be honest, the less prep, pots, pans, utensils, tasks, and cleaning up that are needed, the better. Less mess means less overwhelm.

Knowing which low-effort cooking styles feel easy for you is all you need to keep your ADHD Easy Meal, well, easy.

- **One-pan dinner:** When I need dinner within an hour with no fuss, I throw everything I want onto a baking sheet. Putting everything in one pan is easy on the executive function and takes the least effort possible. For me, this is the easiest way to prepare some of my favorite foods: chicken, potatoes, and carrots. The way you were taught to cook doesn't have to be how you cook as an adult. Sometimes you just don't have the extra energy to peel and chop all the vegetables on chopping boards, separate them into different pans, and season the meats before cooking. You can of course add herbs and spices or marinate the food as you please, but it's nice to know there's nothing wrong with the easiest way when that's all you have space for.

- **Slow cook:** If I want to get dinner out of the way and not think about it later in the day, I turn to my slow cooker. Many slow-cooker recipes call for ingredients that you can get premade or prechopped, so all you have to do is throw everything into it. Since some slow cookers turn off by themselves, you don't even have to track how long the food has been cooking.

- **Blend:** When I need to eat *right now* because I'm late to work, I forgot to eat, or I can't be bothered to turn on the oven, I make my favorite protein shake (more on this shake in "Work with Your Hyperfixations" on page 179).

Some of these styles might be easier for you than others, or what's easiest for you might not be on this list. Maybe your microwave is your best friend or you prefer to assemble whatever is left over in your fridge and call it a meal. At the end of the day, finding what works with your way of being and your lifestyle tends to be what you'll find easiest. And what you find easiest is what will work when you're overwhelmed but still want to eat well at home.

## EATING WELL WHEN EATING OUT

Choosing healthy options when you're at a restaurant can be challenging when you struggle with impulsivity (you forget your goals!) *and* decision-making (so many choices!). Here are some work-arounds if you find yourself always reaching for meals that leave you feeling sluggish for days afterward.

- **Look for protein first:** Scan the menu for your favorite protein-rich foods—roasted or grilled chicken, baked fish, steak, eggs. Or see if it's possible to add an extra protein option if you're having something like a sandwich.

- **Ask for modifications:** Ask to swap the fries for a baked potato or breaded chicken for grilled chicken, or ask to leave the sauce on the side.

- **Order from among the sides:** Order from the sides menu instead of the entrées. I do this a lot for breakfast-type meals so I can build my own healthy plate. I'll ask for three poached eggs with a side of avocado and sourdough toast. I also like how food comes out with nothing touching when you order this way. I don't always want the avocado *on* my toast—I like to fidget with it myself.

- **Use visual aids:** When I'm at a new restaurant, I prefer to see images of the meals I'm considering rather than just reading the descriptions. I'll check the restaurant's Instagram page and look at tagged photos that other customers have posted of its dishes. This allows me to make decisions more quickly, because I have a visual reference of what to expect. By seeing actual photos of the meals, I can also avoid disappointment if the dish doesn't match my expectations based solely on the written description.

- **Honor your sensory needs:** Eating out can be overwhelming when you have sensory sensitivities, and that can lead to comfort eating. It isn't always easy to choose restaurants with quiet atmospheres, so I like to plan visits for the off-peak hours to avoid large crowds, like going out for lunch on a weekday instead of out for dinner on a Saturday night.

## WORK WITH YOUR HYPERFIXATIONS

While I have a rotation of healthy and easy meals that I always find myself going back to, that doesn't mean I make something different every day. My diet looks a little something like this: I eat the same meal every day until I get bored with it. Then I switch to something else and eat *that* until I get bored with it.

Your meals might look similar. Those of us with ADHD tend to intensely fixate on certain things, including specific food combinations and meals. We may eat only a specific food or meal for a while and then move on to a different food or meal, eventually repeating the cycle.

There's nothing wrong with following your food hyper-fixations. It makes shopping easy since you'll automatically know what to add to your shopping cart. It helps you plan meals and reduces the mental load and decision fatigue. It gives you an easy answer when you're wondering what's for dinner.

**A hyperfixation meal is best not just when it makes you feel happy, but also when it helps you thrive.** One of my longest-standing hyperfixation meals is my high-protein shake (see page 168). I've mentioned it a few times already. I've been drinking it almost daily for years and years, and it was one of my staple meals during my transformation after getting diagnosed with ADHD.

It not only tastes like a delicious banana milkshake, but also gives me the many nutrients I need to be and feel healthy, including thirty grams of protein, a mixture of plants (especially because I use a plant-based protein powder), healthy fats from nut butter, plus fiber from a fruit, usually bananas or blueberries. It gives me peace of mind to know that I am getting the nutrients I need, even when I can't be bothered to feed myself. When I get bored, I can change the flavor of the protein powder or switch to a different fruit to make it feel new again, or I'll mix it with oats in the microwave to make a warm, comforting bowl of protein oats. It takes me less than thirty seconds to throw it together, and the process of making it and cleaning the blender doesn't overwhelm me. It's my perfect ADHD Easy Meal, and I can still eat it on repeat and keep reaping the benefits.

On the other hand, repeatedly eating something that your body is giving you negative feedback about will result in gut problems, which can lead to physical and mental health issues. After all, your gut is your "second brain." It can communicate with your actual brain and affect your mood, emotions, and thinking. (We'll explore this more in chapter 7.) Case in point: I took my laptop to a café to do some writing before hitting the gym and sauna. I had the most delicious cheese-and-ham rye bread roll. In fact, it was so delicious that I bought a second one and ate it en route to the gym. *Omg, I could eat this every day forever.* I was already thinking about coming back the next day for more. Within twenty minutes, I had serious belly bloat, discomfort, and heaviness. My drive and motivation dropped, and I had to stop my workout. Into the sauna I went, but I didn't last long there either. Farting in the sauna isn't a good look, and it's not enjoyable for all involved. The message here? If you're going to have a hyperfixation meal, make sure it's something you can tolerate well.

**If you have a hyperfixation meal that makes you feel like crap, but you just can't give it up right now, get creative with how you adapt it.** Maybe keep the most important parts of your favorite meal and swap some of the other components for options that work better for your body. If you know peanut butter irritates your gut, change it to almond butter. If you adore sandwiches but have gluten sensitivity, find a bread you can tolerate. Does going for a walk after eating your hyperfixaton meal help your digestion? If you eat the meal earlier in the day, does that help you avoid an energy crash?

Finally, because it can be hard to eat a variety of foods when you like to eat the same ones on repeat or struggle to introduce new foods into your diet, supplements can help fill any nutritional gaps. Supplements can be a convenient way to get what your body needs, especially when you're too exhausted to think about what you're eating. Even if you eat a balanced diet, they can help ensure you're getting adequate amounts of essential nutrients that modern agricultural practices, soil depletion, food-processing methods, and environmental factors have caused to decline in many foods and that certain medications, such as birth control pills, interfere with the absorption of, leading to nutritional deficiencies. For a list of my go-to supplements, turn to the appendix on page 275. Be sure to consult a healthcare provider before starting any supplement regimen.

**Q:** What if even ADHD Easy Meals are too hard to cook?

**A:** In an ideal world, we would be cooking with fresh vegetables we grow in our own backyard for every meal, but life—and ADHD—don't make this easy. To put it quite frankly, more often than not, you just can't be bothered to chop a vegetable or turn on the stove. Some days, you'll throw a bunch of random things on a plate because you can't muster the energy to cook. You might not have the capacity to function, let alone prep and cook a meal, even an ADHD Easy Meal.

Your goal is to make meals as convenient and ideally as healthy as possible. And that means choosing your battles and knowing when to compromise. While I was writing this sidebar, I was in a hyperfocused state and didn't want to break out of it by switching tasks and cooking. At the same time, I knew I needed healthy food because I hadn't been feeling so great over the past two months. So I ordered takeout, but I chose something that wouldn't make my body feel terrible. On the flip side, a few nights ago I was feeling anxious and had a lot of energy in my head. I needed to do something other than sit and think, so I decided to cook a full meal from scratch. Cooking that meal helped me reconnect to the present moment and to myself. I needed to do that simple act for myself, and I felt so much better afterward.

You can't always do it all. If you're at capacity, you'll need to let an area in your life slide, and that area might be cooking. Other times, cooking might be exactly what you need. **Sometimes we choose what we want, and sometimes we choose what we need.** The more aware we become of moments when we can make this choice, the easier it will be in the future to trust ourselves to know what we need. Instead of feeling bad about ordering takeout, recognize that it was the best option for your well-being *at that moment,* and you made it work as best you could. You're doing your best.

# 7

## Help Your Hormones

*You're not crazy, I promise.*

When I first made the connection between ADHD and hormones, it was because of a seemingly ordinary case of the flu. I was about to go to a yoga class but started feeling flu-like symptoms: a runny nose, a headache, body chills, and a sore throat. I used to rarely get sick, but I was feeling like I was picking up some sort of cold or flu virus each month.

It soon dawned on me that these symptoms appeared during the week before my period and went away when my period started, so I went down another research rabbit hole to see if there was a connection with my cycle. It turned out the flu I was getting the week before my period *wasn't actually a virus at all,* but a form of premenstrual syndrome (PMS). My mind was blown. I'd always understood the signs of PMS to be just a bloated belly and chocolate cravings.

A few months later, things took a turn for the worse. I started having intense emotional breakdowns. Anxiety turned my stomach upside down and left me retching into the toilet. During one particularly bad episode, I crawled into my wardrobe, hoping I could find calm and comfort by being in the small, dark space. It wasn't until a doctor suggested that I might have premenstrual dysphoric disorder (PMDD) that I realized that hormones might be the culprits behind my breakdowns.

I now know firsthand how our hormones play a massive role in every aspect of our well-being. They influence how we think and act daily, as well as our moods, energy level, metabolism, sleep, and sex drive, among many other bodily functions. If you're someone who menstruates, your hormones fluctuate over the course of the month, and these natural fluctuations can worsen your ADHD.

I learned most of what I needed to know about my menstrual cycle in my thirties after deciding to stop using hormonal contraception. Even as an adult, I initially found this information confusing and felt embarrassed that I didn't know this stuff. But ultimately, this knowledge helped me track my cycle, understand why I felt so different from one week to the next, and figure out what I could do to help myself feel my best. I hope it does the same for you. As always, be flexible and curious in your approach to everything you read and learn.

## THE MAJOR PLAYERS: YOUR HORMONES AND ADHD

Hormones are chemical messengers produced by glands in the endocrine system and some organs and tissues. The brain plays an intimate role in regulating these hormones and communicating with other parts of the body to direct them where to go. While there are more than fifty hormones in your body, here are a few of the main players we will focus on in this chapter:

- **Estrogen:** In addition to being one of the key hormones responsible for the development and health of the female reproductive system, menstrual cycle, and other female sexual characteristics, estrogen plays roles in emotional well-being, brain function (including our ability to focus!), the management of blood sugar, collagen production, cholesterol levels, bone strength, skin health, and mood regulation. Estrogen can increase the production or release of dopamine, norepinephrine, and serotonin, the feel-good neurotransmitters that are also crucial for attention, focus, and impulse control. Estrogen is like a vibrant and outgoing friend who brings energy with her wherever she goes. She's the life of the party, always encouraging you to grow beyond your comfort zone, lifting your spirits, and reminding you of how beautiful you are.

- **Progesterone:** Progesterone's main function takes place during ovulation, when it prepares the lining of your uterus for a fertilized egg to potentially implant and grow, but I like to think of it as the "chill" hormone. It aids in pregnancy and lactation, regulates your bleeding when you menstruate, helps improve your mood, and supports thyroid function. Progesterone is the calming and stabilizing friend in your life. She's the one who comes in after estrogen's excitement, bringing a sense of peace and balance. She reminds you to take a step back from the world and relax.

- **Testosterone:** Testosterone is produced by your adrenal glands and ovaries, and it plays pivotal roles in bone strength, sex drive, and ovarian function. Testosterone is the assertive friend who's all about taking charge and getting things done. She never backs down from a challenge and tells you to keep going (sometimes at the cost of your health).

- **Cortisol:** If progesterone is the "chill" hormone, think of cortisol as its opposite. Cortisol is the protective friend who's always on high alert, watching out for threats. In addition to being the hormone responsible for regulating your stress response, cortisol helps control your metabolism and sleep-wake cycle, suppress inflammation, and regulate both blood pressure and blood sugar. This friend has good intentions to keep you safe, but can be a bit overprotective. Spending too much time in her presence can leave you feeling stressed, anxious, and frazzled.

- **Melatonin:** Melatonin governs your sleep-wake cycle, helping to regulate your internal body clock and promoting restful sleep. But its influence goes beyond just ensuring you get a good night's rest. Melatonin also acts as a powerful antioxidant, protecting your cells from damage caused by free radicals. It plays a crucial role in supporting the immune system, promoting overall health and well-being. Melatonin is the reliable friend who ensures you get the rest you need to rejuvenate your body and mind and help you face each day with vitality and resilience.

For many women, the levels of hormones such as estrogen and progesterone fluctuate over the course of a menstrual cycle, which typically lasts twenty-eight days. (In contrast, the hormonal cycle that affects testosterone levels in men lasts only twenty-four hours.) Thanks to our menstrual cycles, our bodies operate according to two internal clocks: circadian rhythms and infradian rhythms. Circadian rhythms run our sleep-wake cycle and affect appetite and digestion. Infradian rhythms are those cycles in the body that last longer than a day, such as the menstrual cycle.

The number of hormonal fluctuations that women experience compared to men has a noticeable impact on our day-to-day well-being. This is especially true for those of us with ADHD—for example, many of us report struggling with heightened PMS symptoms during the luteal phase of our cycle. Understanding the menstrual cycle is important when you have ADHD because hormonal changes throughout your cycle can impact ADHD symptoms like attention, focus, and mood. When you work with your cycle, you can use your knowledge of what's going on in your body to better plan your month and give yourself some compassion and love during the more difficult moments.

## THE THREE PHASES: YOUR PERIOD AND ADHD

You might have noticed that on some days you can get hours and hours of work done and still feel good, whereas on other days it seems like you can't even lift a pen without feeling drained. These changes in your energy level and motivation are connected in part to the three phases of your menstrual cycle. You might have seen references to the *four* phases of the cycle with menstruation as one of the phases, but since menstruation is actually part of the follicular phase, I prefer to keep things simple with three.

- **Follicular phase** (beginning on day one of bleeding and lasting for around fourteen days, until ovulation)

- **Ovulation** (occurring about two weeks after day one of your period and about two weeks before your next bleed; it lasts about one to three days)

- **Luteal phase** (beginning after ovulation and lasting until your next bleed)

Understanding the cyclical nature of your body's hormones will help you live in harmony with your body and the natural ebbing and flowing of your energy levels. I'll discuss how each phase affects how we feel and how we can make changes in our lives to support our bodies and honor our hormones instead of trying to force ourselves to work against our natural rhythms.

## The Follicular Phase

You're in the follicular phase for around two weeks, starting from day one of your period until you ovulate. This is the time when your ovaries prepare an egg for release during ovulation. From day one of your period, estrogen begins a steady climb, boosting your energy, mood, and libido over the following weeks. **Estrogen's positive impact on your feel-good** neurotransmitters is why you might feel as if your mood and energy are heightened when you're in this phase. You're working out more, you feel more motivated and productive, you're sociable and friendly, and you generally feel like the best version of yourself. You might also look leaner because your body is retaining less water, and you're hitting all your personal bests in the gym. Your ADHD-related challenges don't feel as intense as they did two weeks ago. You have more clarity, feel more organized, and are able to regulate your emotions better. You might feel excited about the ideas you have and the new habits you want to start instead of being overwhelmed. This is the best time to try new recipes, plan workouts, and order groceries for the month ahead.

## Ovulation

Ovulation happens about fourteen days after your period starts. Your body releases that carefully prepared egg from a follicle on an ovary and it traverses the fallopian tube, where it waits to give the egg a chance to meet sperm and potentially start a pregnancy. While some women with ADHD feel incredible and at their peak at the time of ovulation, others report experiencing anxiety and intensified ADHD symptoms during these few days, possibly because of the decline in estrogen that accompanies ovulation. Additionally, estrogen has been found to interact with neurotransmitters such as serotonin and GABA in the brain, affecting their balance and contributing to anxiety symptoms.

Personally, I find that I have extra energy during ovulation, and it needs to be used or I end up feeling anxious and irritable. I manage by doing harder workouts and going on longer walks. If you're like me, take advantage of the increased energy level by trying challenging new workouts, exploring new creative activities, and socializing. Use this time to ask for what you want and tackle tasks that require focus, because you may have less energy during your luteal phase. That said, as a general rule of thumb, be mindful of what you say yes to during this time to avoid feeling overwhelmed by a full plate when ovulation passes and your enthusiasm and energy fall. Finally, if you want to get pregnant, this is when you're most fertile.

## The Luteal Phase

The luteal phase is the time between ovulation and your next period. This phase often gets a bad rap because it can be torture for a lot of women. You might literally be fighting for your life. A sharp rise and sudden drop in estrogen during this phase causes your levels of dopamine, serotonin, and norepinephrine to decline, which can worsen executive dys-

**function, impulsivity, and emotional dysregulation.** You might feel more scattered, forgetful, tired, irritable, unmotivated, and sensitive to every sound around you. Your mood may dip, and you might want to retreat, hide from the world, and spend more time alone. While the luteal phase can feel intense and make you feel isolated, it can be a great time to reconnect with yourself and practice a slower way of living.

Stressing yourself out by forcing yourself to perform at the rate you were able to just two weeks prior can do more harm than good. This is because when the body experiences chronic stress, it activates the hypothalamic-pituitary-adrenal (HPA) axis to prioritize cortisol production to cope with the stressor, which can disrupt the normal functioning of other systems and decrease the production of other hormones like progesterone. Now remember, progesterone is our "calming" hormone, and the luteal phase is when our body produces most of it. When your progesterone level is low, it can lead to irregular menstrual periods and make it harder to get pregnant. Additionally, you might experience physical symptoms like bloating, breast tenderness, headaches, and water retention in your arms and legs. These symptoms are often linked to PMS.

## PMS & PMDD & ADHD

Women with ADHD often experience more severe symptoms of premenstrual syndrome (PMS) than women without it, and 46 percent of us are affected by PMDD. PMS symptoms can range from cramps, bloating, and digestive problems to noise sensitivity, worsening of allergy symptoms, and fatigue.

PMDD, on the other hand, is a more extreme form of PMS that usually involves profound anxiety, deep depression, severe mood swings, and suicidal thoughts. PMDD can make life unbearable and significantly interfere with relationships, work, school, and social activities. Women with PMDD report experiencing extreme sensitivity to rejection, more emotional meltdowns, and intrusive thoughts, and they are at an increased risk of attempting suicide. You might feel like an entirely different person and have the impulse to uproot your entire life, quit your job, move to another country, or get a divorce—only to feel completely normal a week later when your period starts.

Both PMS and PMDD are signals that something is not working right in the body, leaving those affected by them with an abnormal sensitivity to the body's natural hormonal fluctuations. Specifically, **PMDD is actually thought to be a severe sensitivity in the brain to the normal rise and fall of hormones during the luteal phase of the menstrual cycle.** You could think of it as a miscommunication between the brain and hormones. Chronic stress, unprocessed emotions, and trauma can all play a role in developing PMDD. These include adverse childhood experiences such as chronic household dysfunction and abuse. For example, in one study, 85 percent of women with PMDD were found to have experienced early life trauma, with 71 percent of those women experiencing emotional abuse.

Experiencing intense physical and emotional pain before a period has become expected, but that doesn't mean it should be normal. If you've spoken to a doctor about any PMS or PMDD symptoms, my hope would be that they can help you understand how your cycle impacts the way you're feeling.*

## RETURN TO THE BASICS

If you want to feel healthy and happy, being in flow with your cycle and managing hormonal imbalances whenever possible is a massive piece of the puzzle. You can do a lot to manage your monthly luteal lows, reduce the intensity of what you

---

* Unfortunately, this isn't always the case. Many primary care physicians lack training in female hormone conditions like PMDD, leading to misdiagnoses. There's no blood test to confirm it, and hormone tests can come back normal. If the psychological symptoms are taken in isolation, they can be mistaken for generalized anxiety or clinical depression.

experience during your cycles, and help yourself function better from day to day.

Supporting your body isn't about thinking up some unrealistic practices, but about returning to the basics, a lot of which you already know deep down you should do or might even already be doing since you've read the previous chapters. Here are five ideas that will give you a good start on supporting and optimizing your hormone system's function.

## Track Your Cycle

When I stopped taking oral contraceptive pills, I started using an app[*] that helps me track my cycle and shows me where in my cycle I am as my form of birth control. The app I use is an FDA-approved birth control method that allows me to avoid pregnancy by letting me know exactly when I can get pregnant and when I can't. Beyond helping me avoid pregnancy, the app has helped me live more in tune with my body as a whole. Before, I used to wake up surprised to find that my period had arrived. Sometimes I'd get a scare, wondering if my period was late, and frantically try to remember

---

[*] The app I use is called Natural Cycles, but there are plenty of great options out there for you to choose from. Period-tracking apps collect personal data about your cycle, so if privacy is a concern for you, be sure to check their privacy policies.

when the last one was. I'd check email receipts to see when I last ordered tampons, or check my phone's photo album to try to find a photo of me in that outfit I remembered wearing during my last period.

With the app, I was able to track when I was ovulating and could get pregnant, and when I wasn't ovulating and wouldn't get pregnant. For the first time in my life, I could see why I had more energy right after my period but lacked energy the week before my period. I had never paid attention to ovulation. I hadn't noticed the way my body was on a hormonal clock and how those hormones affected how I felt from one week to the next.

Tracking your cycle will give you crucial insights into your body and mind. And it's easier than ever. There are so many period-tracking apps, including some that are FDA approved as birth control methods using a regulated medical device. Many of these apps sync with wearable fitness trackers, making it easier than ever to know where you are in your cycle. Then you can draw on your other healthy habits to deal with your experience of the different phases accordingly. Think of tracking your cycle as a foundation that you can use to build the rest of your habits on. The more difficult phases of your cycle may still be challenging, but by practicing healthy habits, they will become manageable. In fact, it's always during the luteal phase that I remember how powerful my habits are, because my symptoms are most intense when I'm not following them.

## HORMONAL CONTRACEPTION

Hormonal birth control works by releasing *synthetic* hormones that mimic natural estrogen and progesterone to trick your body into thinking it's already pregnant. This stops ovulation and leads you to experience a "withdrawal bleed" that looks exactly like a regular period. For some of us, these synthetic hormones can negatively affect how our bodies later produce our naturally occurring hormones.

Here's where the negative effects often begin: Many synthetic versions of progesterone, called progestins, are made from testosterone. Though they're meant to mimic natural progesterone, they are structurally similar to testosterone and don't bind to progesterone receptors as well as your naturally produced progesterone does. These progestins don't bind only to the progesterone receptors; they also attach to other receptors, like those of testosterone and cortisol. When a synthetic hormone binds to the wrong receptor, it can send incorrect signals and disrupt the body's balance, leading to unpleasant side effects. A 2023 study found that women with ADHD already have a three times higher risk of developing depression. But women who have ADHD and take oral contraceptives—also known as "the Pill"—have a *six times* higher risk of developing depression compared to women without ADHD taking the same pill.

Even after you stop taking the Pill, it might take several

months to rebalance your natural hormones. Some women experience mood swings, anxiety, and depression after stopping hormonal birth control, known as "post–birth control syndrome." Personally, I never suffered PMS or PMDD before going on the birth control pill, but when I stopped it after six years, I began experiencing these symptoms. Perhaps my body struggled to readjust after metabolizing synthetic hormones for so long.

The point here isn't to dissuade you from taking birth control. I started using it at age twenty-five for its sheer convenience, so I get it. But I do believe many of us stroll into the doctor's office and opt in to taking the Pill without having any real context on what it actually does to our bodies, or without looking at other options. I'd like to encourage you to do some research before deciding what's right for you. Dr. Sarah E. Hill's *How the Pill Changes Everything* is a great resource for collecting more detailed information. You can also discuss nonhormonal birth control options with a healthcare provider, and if you find that staying on the Pill works best for you, sometimes a simple change in the dosage or type of birth control can improve side effects. Keep tabs on your mood and any side effects when starting a new method. Watch out for prescription cascades, where one medication's side effects are then treated with another.

At the end of the day, you know what the right decision for your body and your lifestyle is. My hope is that you will take this information and use it to better inform your decision before making it. What works for you may not work for others.

## Feed Your Gut Microbiome

The gut microbiome contains trillions of tiny organisms like bacteria, fungi, viruses, and even parasites that live in your digestive system, forming a community that plays essential roles in digestion, immune function (70 to 80 percent of your immune cells are located in the gut!), metabolism, mental health, the nervous system, and hormonal health. It wields this much influence because your gut has a close neurological link with the brain, with the two using a network of hundreds of millions of neurons and the vagus nerve to send and receive messages. This is called the gut-brain axis.

Most important for what we're discussing in this chapter is that the microbiome plays a big role in your hormone balance. It helps with things like breaking down food and absorbing nutrients that help build hormones, communicating with your brain (like we just discussed), and reducing inflammation to improve hormone production and signaling. For example, there is a community of bacteria known as the estrobolome in your gut microbiome. They play a crucial role in managing estrogen, which is produced primarily in your ovaries and sent throughout your body to act on other tissues and organs. Eventually, that active estrogen gets filtered through the liver, which deactivates it and then sends it off to your gut. If the gut is working right, most of that deactivated estrogen gets excreted in your stool.

Sadly, your gut microbiome can't do its job in unhealthy conditions, like when you are chronically stressed, consuming lots of ultra-processed foods and alcohol, and regularly using medications like antibiotics. Rather than nourishing it, these conditions have left your gut microbiome starved of the nutrients it needs (such as fiber, vitamins, minerals, and phytochemicals) to help keep you healthy. This can allow unfriendly gut bacteria to grow. Some types of unfriendly gut bacteria can actually *reactivate* inactive estrogen, causing excess estrogen to rise. While estrogen can positively influence dopamine levels, as discussed earlier, too much estrogen, referred to as "estrogen dominance," can disrupt neurotransmitter balance and adversely affect mood, cognition, and emotional regulation. In addition, estrogen dominance can lead to a range of health issues, including autoimmune disease, polycystic ovary syndrome (PCOS), and even breast cancer.

A healthy microbiome is diverse. To maintain this diversity, aim to incorporate a wide array of plants (see "Eat More

Plants" on page 171) and colors into your meals. By diversi-
fying your plant intake, you'll be supplying your body with
many different essential nutrients, fiber, and combinations
of antioxidants and vitamins crucial for nurturing your gut.
Each color of plant foods contains different phytochemicals,
which nourish different types of beneficial bacteria in your
gut. For example, red, yellow, and green peppers each contain different phytochemicals even though they are techni-
cally the same vegetable. Eating a variety of plants of
different colors is like building different houses for different
microorganisms.

## Eat Fats

It's well known now that decades ago, large food companies
paid researchers to play down the link between sugar intake
and health problems in the media and to make *fats* the enemy
instead. The eighties' and nineties' trends of emphasizing
low-fat foods and demonizing healthy fats has left generations of women afraid of this important macronutrient that
can help with our hormone-related health problems.

Specifically, in addition to other health benefits like helping balance your blood sugar, eating healthy fats like the
omega-3s found in fatty fish supports hormone production.
Omega-3 fats are able to do this by keeping cell walls strong,
especially in hormone-producing glands like the adrenals and

ovaries. Strong cell walls help hormones work properly by ensuring the right signals get through to the cells. Since your brain is made of mostly fat (about 60 percent), it relies on these fats for optimal function and protection. **Omega-3 fatty acids, in particular, play a key role in brain health by reducing inflammation and supporting brain function. They enhance how neurons communicate with one another and smooth the communication between them, which can help your brain better regulate hormone levels. By taking in more omega-3s from healthy fat sources, you can potentially avoid the miscommunication problems that could contribute to conditions like PMDD.**

Today, with our modern-day diets, we're eating too many omega-6 fats and not enough omega-3 fats. Researchers suggest that human beings evolved on a diet with a ratio of omega-6 to omega-3 of approximately 1:1, whereas in Western diets today the ratio is closer to 15:1. For example, omega-6s are found in popular everyday seed oils like canola/ rapeseed, soybean, and sunflower oil, which are common in a lot of ultra-processed foods. If we aren't careful about checking the ingredients of our foods, and even some of the supplements we're taking daily, we could be pumping extra omega-6s into us. Having too much omega-6 fats can stir up inflammation, which messes with your hormones; on the other hand, omega-3 fatty acids help to counteract inflammation, promoting hormone balance and supporting overall health. You can increase your omega-3 intake by eating foods such as salmon, sardines, mackerel, herring, anchovies, chia seeds, flaxseeds, walnuts, spirulina, pasture-raised eggs, and grass-fed meat.*

If you don't eat fish or meat, keep in mind that plant-based omega-3 sources like flaxseed, chia seeds, and hemp seeds are more difficult for your bodies to use for brain health and inflammation reduction. To support this conversion, try including foods that are good sources of methylated B vitamins and magnesium, such as spinach. You could also take an algae-based omega-3 supplement, which is the primary source of omega-3s in the ocean food chain.

## Practice Food Timing

A lot of us, ADHD women especially, are wreaking havoc on our hormones by having inconsistent mealtimes. We don't eat all day, then maybe we'll eat a huge meal at night and can't sleep because digesting the large meal interrupts the release of the sleep hormone melatonin. Even when we do manage to fall asleep, our body is unable to get the quality shut-eye we need to feel fueled and energized the next morning, further disrupting our hormones.

---

* Wild-caught fish, grass-fed meat, and pasture-raised eggs typically have higher omega-3 content and fewer omega-6 fats than their farmed alternatives. This is because wild-caught, grass-fed, and pasture-raised animals consume foods that are closer to their natural diets, which are higher in omega-3s than the grains that are usually fed to farmed animals.

Food timing can get our mealtimes back on track. I got sold on the concept after I listened to a podcast episode on longevity by David Sinclair, PhD. What surprised me was what he shared about a study investigating intermittent fasting that was conducted on a few groups of mice. Long story short, the mice that lived the longest out of all the groups were fed within a window of time that matched their circadian rhythm. They didn't just live longer—they lived 34 percent longer compared to the control group. We're not mice, and studies of this sort haven't been done on humans yet, but the episode sparked my curiosity enough to make me question my own eating habits. The idea that food timing can help us live in sync with one of our internal clocks felt like common sense and something that we've forgotten to do over the years.

I was someone who grazed all day until right before bed, but right there and then, I chose to give it a shot and changed the times I eat my first and last meals of the day. In fact, I like to think of intermittent fasting simply as *food timing*, as we're simply timing when we eat to enhance how we feel. Tweaking the times I ate made me feel incredible. Within a few days, my energy, mood, and focus went through the roof. I found it so easy to eat well, be well, and live well. I lost a lot of inflammation and puffiness from my face and body, and extra fat was dropping off me with ease, without me needing to increase my workouts or restrict my favorite foods.

After feeling the benefits of more clarity and energy, I dived into finding out why and how the timing of food and fasting helps those with ADHD. While there hasn't been much research done on the specific impacts of food timing on ADHD, food timing can enhance brain function in a number of ways that could help lessen your ADHD symptoms. First, it increases levels of BDNF (brain-derived neurotrophic factor), which supports new brain cell growth and improves memory, supports metabolic health, and helps to stabilize blood sugar levels, thus improving insulin sensitivity. It also gives your body enough time to digest food *before* sleeping, so it can direct more of its energy to renewal and repair during sleep. Eating close to bedtime can throw off the body's internal clock. Your body prioritizes the release of insulin, which can prevent melatonin from being released on time. You may find yourself more awake and with more energy at night.

Eating this way not only helps control cravings, mood swings, and energy surges and crashes but can also boost the repair and renewal of cells through a process known as autophagy. Autophagy involves breaking down and repurposing old or damaged parts of cells, which reduces inflammation and lowers the risk of diseases. And, because the basic principle is "Eat only during your chosen eating window," it's straightforward and doesn't strain your executive function because there's no need to keep track of what you eat and when you eat it.

When selecting a window, a common option that people often recommend is to eat over the course of eight hours a day and fast for the remaining sixteen hours. But you can keep food timing even simpler with this one guideline: **Have your last meal before the sun goes down or three hours before sleeping.** I do the latter during the winter, as it gets dark as early as 3:00 P.M.

If you tried what's known as "intermittent fasting" before but felt that it left you moody, shaky, and unhappy, you might have taken fasting advice without keeping your hormone fluctuations in mind. While you can use the rule of thumb of stopping eating three hours before bed at any point in your cycle, other rules around food timing—specifically, when you have your first meal of the day—become a bit more complicated when you take your hormones into account. As a woman who menstruates, you can't fast or treat your body in the same way every day to feel at optimal health. In other words, you can't fast like a man.

Keep these hormone-centric tips in mind:

- During the follicular phase (from the start of your period to ovulation), when estrogen levels rise, you can tolerate longer fasting periods. This is when you can do the popular 16:8 method we briefly discussed earlier, which means eating during an eight-hour window each day and giving your body about sixteen hours (or more) to rest and repair. To be clear, when you're doing this, it doesn't mean you're skipping meals. You're simply delaying your breakfast with a meal rich in protein, fats, and fiber, and eating your dinner earlier than usual.

- During ovulation and into the luteal phase, eat within an hour of waking up. Going without food for an extended period of time may put your body into a stress response, which can negatively affect the production of progesterone, increasing the severity of PMS and worsening your ADHD symptoms, as discussed earlier. During this time, it's important to listen to your body and be flexible with your diet. For example, you might notice your body craves more carbohydrates during this time—this is normal, your body is designed to crave them! If you're used to having a breakfast rich in protein and fats (eggs and avocado, for example), think about adding some carbohydrates to your plate during this time in your cycle (a sweet potato, a banana, or quinoa is a great option in the luteal phase).

On a deeper level, when we practice food timing with our internal clocks in mind, we get back in touch with our body's natural rhythm and way of living. The body is so intelligent, but we live in complete opposition to it a lot of the time. Setting up a three-hour cushion of digestion before bed and being flexible about food timing during the luteal phase are simple steps toward listening to this intelligence.

## Swap Hormone-Disrupting Products

Unfortunately, we may be using many products in our everyday lives that throw off our endocrine system. Many of them, from the plastic bottles we drink from to the products we wash with and the perfume we spray on ourselves, contain endocrine-disrupting chemicals (EDCs), such as phthalates, BPA (bisphenol A), pesticides, heavy metals, and PFAS (per- and polyfluoroaklyl substances, often referred to as forever chemicals). EDCs have been linked to a wide range of health issues, such as endometriosis, PCOS, irregular periods, early puberty, cancer, and infertility, as well as neurological and learning disabilities. EDCs can also mess with the way neurotransmitters like dopamine and norepinephrine work. This can throw off how the brain controls attention, mood, and behavior, which is already challenging when you have ADHD.

So, what are EDCs? They are chemicals or mixtures of chemicals that interfere with the way our hormones work. They mess with your ovaries' ability to produce estrogen and progesterone. By stopping our *actual* hormones from doing their job, EDCs can cause problems with fertility, induce hormone sensitive cancers, and contribute to obesity,

**among other effects.** For example, BPA, found primarily in plastics, has been shown to bind to estrogen receptors and mess up the way our cells communicate with one another. Endocrine disrupters, by imitating or obstructing hormone functioning, can interfere with the body's detoxification pathways, slowing down the elimination of waste products and resulting in a buildup of harmful substances. This increased toxic burden can contribute to various diseases.

Other research has shown that there is a connection between EDCs and ADHD. "Endocrine-disrupting chemicals present in our food, air, water, and personal products may cause cognitive-behavioral disorders like attention-deficit/hyperactivity disorder or overeating in future generations," explained Emily N. Hilz, PhD, a postdoctoral fellow at the University of Texas at Austin. One 2020 study found that exposure to common phthalates, which are found in beauty products, cleaning products, food packaging, building materials, toys, and fragrances, during the adolescent years may be "associated with behaviors characteristic of ADHD." Another study, from 2018, found that moms who were exposed to phthalates during pregnancy had a higher likelihood of having children with ADHD.

Phthalates aren't the only EDCs linked to ADHD. Pregnant women who used diethylstilbestrol, a synthetic estrogen that was once commonly prescribed to prevent pregnancy complications, had an increased risk of future generations of their families having ADHD. The grandchildren of women who took diethylstilbestrol were found to be 36 percent more likely to have ADHD than the grandchildren of women who did not. This drug, which has been associated with "multi-generational neurodevelopmental deficits" was prescribed to millions of pregnant women for decades. Your mother or grandmother might very well have taken the drug while pregnant, possibly affecting the way your brain developed all these years later.

Not all of the chemicals we interact with on a daily basis are endocrine disrupters, but we also haven't studied many of them for their long-term effects on human health. More than eighty thousand synthetic chemicals have entered our food, air, water, and personal care products over the last fifty years, almost none of which have been tested for their combined impact on human health. According to the Environmental Working Group, the average person applies nine personal care products to their body daily, containing 126 unique ingredients. You might think "Not me, I don't wear makeup," but think about even the most basic daily products: toothpaste, deodorant, shampoo, perfume, lip balm, hand soap, sunscreen, body lotion. The number of products is easy to rack up, even if you're someone who doesn't wear much makeup. These few products alone can contain hundreds of unique ingredients, many of which are endocrine disrupters. And that's before we even consider household products.

*EDCs are everywhere.* Finding out that many of the family's favorite household products might hurt our health even though they have been on shelves *for decades* hits hard.

I've heard some people argue against worrying about EDCs: "There are bad chemicals in everything"; "We can't live in bubble wrap"; "It's only a tiny bit. It won't kill you." I used to believe the same, and while they're right that we can't live entirely risk-free or change the world overnight, I argue that it all adds up, and it's worth making our homes as healthy as we can and choosing better-for-us products, especially because women like us with ADHD are more sensitive to hormonal changes.

This doesn't mean that I panic and stress myself out about avoiding exposure to all EDCs. Instead, I choose my battles (and my poisons, to put it bluntly) because sometimes I forget, sometimes EDC-free options aren't accessible, and sometimes I just don't have the capacity to think about them.

If you're looking for how to begin reducing the number of EDCs in your life, here are some of the swaps that can make the most difference:

- **Start with the products you use *the most*:** Make switches in your everyday products, such as deodorant, shampoo, face wash, and lip balm, to cleaner alternatives. One of the easier swaps I suggest to those just starting out is opting for a mineral-based sunscreen over a chemical sunscreen. You can also make a huge difference by simply ditching the things you don't *really* need, like the air freshener hanging in your car and the laundry fabric softener. You don't need to overhaul your entire life for your swaps to have a big impact. Have a couple of go-to brands you can rely on for multiple products, such as beauty brands that have labels indicating they are free of parabens, phthalates, or sulfates.

- **Dump the bleach-based cleaning products:** I now have an all-purpose kitchen cleaner, a bathroom cleaner, a floor cleaner, and a glass and mirror cleaner that I order online from a company that produces safe, nontoxic products free of EDCs. I have my products autoshipped to me every two months to make life easier for my ADHD brain.

- **Reduce plastic for use in food storage:** Don't heat food in plastic containers or drink hot beverages from plastic glasses to prevent the EDCs in the plastic from leaching into your food. This is especially common when we heat frozen foods and takeout orders. Even if your plastic container is marked "microwave safe," the designation only means that the plastic won't outright melt. To be truly safe, always transfer your food onto a glass or ceramic plate before microwaving. A lot of food is sold in plastic, so it's not always easy to make the switch, but you might find a choice of glass instead of plastic packaging more common in some foods such as nut butters and condiments such as mayonnaise.

- **Reduce your exposure to PFAS:** PFAS, also called forever chemicals, can remain in the body for many years, gradually accumulating and potentially causing health issues over time. Known for their water- and stain-repellent properties, PFAS are commonly found in nonstick cookware, food packaging, waterproof clothing, and even sweat-resistant gym wear, such as leggings. To reduce my exposure, I've switched to wearing more loose-fitting clothes made from cotton or linen blends when I'm not working out, and when buying new cookware I opt for stainless steel where possible.

- **Break up with those car and home air fresheners, scented candles, and perfumes:** Have you ever seen "fragrance" listed on an ingredients label? Manufacturers aren't required to reveal the ingredients in a fragrance when it's used in products like air fresheners, candles, and perfumes. They can simply label it as "fragrance," even if it contains thirty different synthetic compounds. Fragrances are combinations of chemicals used to create pleasant scents in products such as perfumes. Cleaning products, detergents, fabric softeners, air fresheners, and deodorants also commonly contain harmful chemi-

cals added as fragrances and are among the most common endocrine-disrupting chemicals. To freshen your
home, keep your windows open to let air circulate, and
use fragrant fresh flowers and plants for a pleasant scent.
If you can't give up perfume, look for those with natural
essential oils and botanical extracts, or reduce how often
you wear them and how much you use.

• **Use organic tampons and pads:** Many conventional
tampons and pads are made from viscose, also known as
rayon, which is made from wood pulp. While it is de-
rived from wood pulp, the process of converting wood
pulp into viscose typically involves the use of toxic
chemicals. Viscose is used in tampons because it is
highly absorbent. However, concerns have been raised
about the possibility of chemical residues remaining in
the final product. The lining of the vagina is sensitive
and can easily absorb harmful substances that may be in
our period and feminine hygiene products. To avoid potential exposure to harmful chemicals, tampons and
pads made from 100 percent organic cotton can be a
safer choice. Organic cotton is grown, processed, and
harvested completely differently from conventional cotton, without harmful pesticides or fertilizers.

If all of these swaps aren't realistic for your lifestyle right
now, don't worry. As with everything else in this book, you can

do what you can, when you can—it's okay to start small. These tiny efforts *do* make a difference and add up over time. In fact, a scientific study found that *in just twenty-eight days,* women who stopped using personal care products with parabens and phthalates had positive cellular changes in their breast tissue, potentially reversing some cancer-related cell behaviors.

## Stress Kills Your Hormone Balance

There's nothing like a bout of stress to really send your hormones into a frenzy. As explained in the discussion of the luteal phase, excessive stress affects the hypothalamic-pituitary-adrenal (HPA) axis, which regulates the body's stress response. In times of persistent stress, the HPA axis may overactivate, leading to sustained high levels of our main stress hormone, cortisol. This can disrupt the functioning of other hormones, such as estrogen and progesterone. While cortisol doesn't directly lower estrogen and progesterone levels, it can interfere with their production and function. For example, cortisol can affect how estrogen and progesterone bind to their receptors. So, even if estrogen and progesterone levels stay relatively normal, their ability to function may be compromised when cortisol levels are high, contributing to disruptions in the menstrual cycle. Prolonged stress can also affect other parts of the endocrine system by decreasing thyroid function and insulin sensitivity, weakening the immune system, and increasing the risk of autoimmune diseases.

But here's the thing: The chaos that stress causes doesn't stop there. Long-term stress also invites its friend testosterone to join in. Women normally produce the small amounts of testosterone that we need, but when testosterone levels are too high for too long, they may begin to experience irregular cycles, excess hair growth, acne, and mood and fertility issues. High testosterone levels are also closely associated with conditions like PCOS.

One of the most basic ways we can reduce stress is, again, to live in alignment with what our bodies need. I used to wonder why I felt anxious, unmotivated, and depressed before my period. Even though my body needed quiet, slow, sleepy downtime for a few days, I fought it and forced myself to perform. I was fueled by the need to keep being productive at all costs. I bought into the lie that strong, independent women don't need to slow down. And even when I did slow down and take breaks from work, in the background of my mind there was a constant stressful buzz because I was afraid of falling behind. Underneath it all, I had this deep-seated feeling that I needed to fill every spare crack of time with more work. I thought hormonal fluctuations weren't an excuse to be at less than my best and that I was supposed to be productive every day. But productivity isn't a measure of self-worth, and your best self isn't necessarily your most productive self. When we suppress our bodies' needs and deny them rest and nurturing, they will react badly. We need to surrender to rest, give ourselves space to sometimes live slowly, change how we respond to stress, and set boundaries with others. We need to reconnect to our emotions and natural way of being—and not just for our hormone health, but also for our sanity.

---

*Productivity isn't a measure of self-worth, and your best self isn't necessarily your most productive self.*

---

**Q:** I feel embarrassed and find it hard to cut myself some slack when my cycle affects my ADHD, even though I don't feel my best. What do I do about these conflicting feelings?

**A:** You're not the only one who feels this way. I see the same tendency with new coaching clients who tell me, "Last week I was so motivated and this week I'm not. I don't know what's wrong with me; I must be doing it wrong?!" During the ten days before my period, I also see myself in a harsher light. I'm self-critical, judgmental, and less sensitive with myself, even though I know it's only me who sees the problems.

The next time you feel this way, practicing self-compassion, as we discussed in chapter 2, will help you tame this self-criticism. Try asking yourself where you are in your cycle and remind yourself that you're having a normal reaction to the way your body works. Your hormones affect everything, and your hormone levels change every day. These fluctuations don't mean you only have the ability to exercise during one week of the month; they simply mean you need to give yourself flexibility. For example, if you run every day, it's okay for the speed and intensity of the runs to vary throughout the month.

Your body telling you that it's in pain, is tired, or needs rest isn't an invitation for you to say, "Wanna bet?" and prove it wrong. You cannot force yourself to work against your natural cycle, and recognizing when to take it easy will also help you avoid hormone imbalances, fatigue, and burnout. It's okay to be gentle, to go slower, rest more, and start to get into sync with the flow you were born with. If you lean into the feelings, work around them, honor them, and give your body what it needs, you'll find your PMS symptoms might lessen, your luteal phase will stop feeling so bad, and your body won't need to scream anymore for you to hear it.

# 8

.

# Regulate Your Nervous System and Reconnect

*We're dysregulated,*
*and it's making our ADHD worse.*

Remember that year in my life when I was having intense emotional breakdowns? Well, it was during this period when I decided to do something I often did when feeling unstable—make a drastic life change and leave my future self to deal with the consequences of my impulsive decisions.

In the space of two weeks, I cut my hair off, dyed it black, packed up the home that I loved, got in a car with Ruairí, and drove to Spain with no hotels booked. Sounds like a dream, right? Wrong. The stress of the move, the sadness of leaving my home, and the challenge of navigating a new country with all our stuff and our dog in the back of the car—plus a huge work deadline—was more than I could handle.

After ten weeks of living on the road, I broke down in tears at the kitchen table in our Airbnb. I missed London, my home, my routine, all the little rituals of my days that kept me grounded, healthy, and happy. I wasn't able to write or work because I was so all over the place. My energy was scattered, and it was at this moment that I realized what I'd been saying about hating routines wasn't true. It's routine that keeps me sane. I *need* routine. We drove back to London and after a few more months of staying in Airbnbs and hotels, and wasting a lot of money, we found a home. But after just twenty-four hours, we realized we had been sold a nightmare. A battle with the landlord began, which caused further dysregulation, overwhelm, and panic attacks. I was not okay. I woke up crying and went to sleep crying. It felt like if *one* more thing happened, I wouldn't want to be on this earth anymore.

Writing about this experience now saddens me, because I didn't want to hurt myself. I was just so overwhelmed at the time that I couldn't see, think, or feel clearly, and I had so much secret shame because I couldn't understand why I couldn't just "handle it" like I always had in the past. I felt as if my body had been hijacked and I was operating in survival mode, a mere shell of myself. I realized that no amount of protein and running was going to fix this.

Relief finally came on my birthday that summer, after an early-morning appointment with my therapist, who had trained as a doctor before opening her therapy practice. Going beyond talk therapy, she drew on her medical training and explained how my biology was out of balance and my nervous system was dysregulated, causing all this overwhelm. In fact, a number of studies have found evidence of nervous system dysregulation in patients with PMDD. She gave me hope by reminding me that the hopelessness I was feeling made sense for the emergency state my nervous system was in, and that with the right tools, I had the power to move out of this state and into one of healing, relaxation, and calm.

It was during this period of my life that I had an aha moment: *Oh my God. It's all nervous system work.* Gabor Maté, MD, believes ADHD is "rooted in multi-generational family stress and in disturbed social conditions in a stressed society." And to be totally honest, when I first came across his research in 2021, I didn't want to believe him, because I was put off by his explanation of ADHD. But as I started working on regulating my own nervous system, the more a lot of my ADHD and PMDD symptoms lessened in severity.

So many of us with ADHD are severely overwhelmed, a state that often stems from having a dysregulated nervous system. We're disconnected from ourselves, and lack exposure to natural light and nature, movement, and the minerals and vitamins in wholesome foods. We're carrying years of trauma, hiding stress and shame, bottling up our emotions, consuming too much alcohol, sleeping poorly, overextending ourselves, living on social media—all of this is making us sick. External factors like mold exposure and toxin overload also contribute to the problem, leaving our bodies in states of imbalance, dysregulation, and distress. Reconnecting with who we are and regulating our nervous system can not only improve our ADHD symptoms, but also lead us back to a state of health and happiness. If we come back to ourselves, we will feel better.

## SURVIVAL MODE DISCONNECTS YOU FROM YOURSELF

When you're dehydrated, undernourished, running on no sleep, glued to your phone notifications, reacting to every trigger, breathing shallow and fast, and running late with unfinished tasks scattered everywhere, of course you're going to be a cranky, hot mess. When you live like this on repeat, you are sending your body into emergency mode and knocking it out of homeostasis, which disrupts the functioning of your nervous system. An out-of-whack nervous system can blur your sense of self and spark a cascade of reactions in the body, which can lead to chronic health problems over time.

### How Regulated Turns into Dysregulated

The autonomic nervous system is the control system that manages bodily functions you don't have to think about, like your heartbeat and digestion. It can also affect conscious thought and decision-making processes.

The autonomic nervous system has two parts that work together:

- The **sympathetic nervous system** helps your body react to a threat or danger by preparing it for action through the "fight or flight" response. It's why you sweat, breathe shallowly, and feel like your heart is beating out of your chest when you're freaking out. It revs up your body to help you deal with whatever challenge comes your way, getting you ready to fight or flee in a flash.

- The **parasympathetic nervous system** helps your body relax and unwind after a stressful situation through the "rest and digest" response. So when you're done dealing with a threat or danger, this system kicks in to slow down your heart rate, calm your breathing, and promote digestion, giving your body a chance to rest and recover and leaving you feeling relaxed and grounded.

When your nervous system is regulated, your body can effectively handle stress and return to a calm state afterward, moving between states of tension and relaxation easily. You can take on life's daily challenges without feeling overwhelmed, balancing the vigilance of the sympathetic nervous system and the relaxation of the parasympathetic nervous system. Having a regulated nervous system doesn't mean you're always passive, calm, or happy, but that you can move between the two states with ease. This can help us stay mentally clear, emotionally stable, and physically healthy.

**The most common dysregulated state that ADHD women often find themselves in is one of sympathetic hyperarousal—when the body remains in a prolonged state of heightened alertness due to the continuous activation of the fight-or-flight response.** When the nervous system is in this state, it tends to prioritize immediate survival responses over cognitive functions. Because your brain is mostly focused on perceived threats, it becomes even more difficult to concentrate on tasks, regulate emotions, and make thoughtful decisions. You may feel more impulsive and easily distracted, and experience more anxiety and mood swings. You're less able to navigate the ups and downs of life, and you become physically and emotionally sensitive to even the smallest stressors in your environment. Think of it like your body's alarm system going off too often, even when there's no real danger.

So, how did we get here? What happened to make us dysregulated in the first place? An imbalanced nervous system can result from a mix of various factors, including chronic stress, trauma, environmental influences, and lifestyle choices. These factors can contribute to disconnecting from yourself and disrupt the normal functioning of your nervous system. Some of the key contributing factors include:

- **Circadian rhythms:** When we throw off our circadian rhythms, we throw off our nervous system and make it less able to cope with stress. We've been working against our inner clocks since lightbulbs were invented in 1879. It's common knowledge that blue light from our screens is making it harder for us to fall asleep by hurting the body's natural ability to release melatonin, the sleep hormone that your brain produces in response to darkness.

- **Lifestyle factors:** Among these are a poor diet and deficiencies in nutrients such as B vitamins, vitamin D, calcium, amino acids, zinc, potassium, and magnesium; a sedentary lifestyle; poor-quality sleep; ongoing stress; dependency on caffeine, alcohol, and certain medications; and exposure to environmental toxins such as heavy metals, pesticides, molds, and endocrine-disrupting chemicals. Mineral deficiencies are often overlooked. For example, our adrenal glands use a lot of minerals to manage stress, including electrolytes and trace minerals. Electrolytes, such as sodium, potassium, calcium, and magnesium, are a type of mineral that carries an electric charge and is crucial for maintaining fluid balance, transmitting nerve signals, and regulating muscle function. Trace minerals, such as iron, zinc, selenium, and copper, are required in smaller amounts, play vital roles in enzyme function, hormone production, and immune response.

- **Low vagal tone:** The longest cranial nerves in the body are the two vagus nerves, and they run down our left and right sides from our brain to our colon. One of their jobs is to disengage your sympathetic nervous system to bring your body back to a resting state. We measure how well the vagus nerves are functioning through vagal tone. When vagal tone is low, it means that the vagus nerve is less effective in regulating stress responses and other bodily functions like breathing and digestion. Low vagal tone has been linked with ADHD. ADHDers may spend more time in a state of fight or flight and experience more chronic stress, which can lead to even lower vagal tone over time.[*]

- **Unfinished stress responses:** An unfinished stress response happens when your body starts the physiological

---

[*] If you're curious about your vagal tone, you can track it at home by checking your heart rate variability (HRV), a functionality that a lot of health and fitness trackers have today. Check your ring or watch to see if you can track HRV. The higher the HRV, the lower the stress level and the better your nervous system health. Spoiler: Those of us with ADHD and a dysregulated nervous system tend to have low HRV.

process of responding to stress but doesn't complete it. This can happen when the stressor isn't fully resolved or you don't adequately process the stress; perhaps you pushed down your distress, hid it away, and pretended you were fine. For example, if you felt threatened as a child, your nervous system would have initiated a fight-or-flight response. But if you were unable to actually complete that response by fighting back or escaping the scary situation, you might freeze, "playing dead" to avoid being targeted. If you don't release this built-up energy through shaking and trembling, the trapped energy signals the ongoing threat to the body. This unfinished business can imprint on your nervous system and cause you to get stuck in a stress response.

- **Childhood trauma:** Traumatic experiences in childhood such as emotional neglect, verbal abuse, or witnessing violence can alter the way our brain processes information and regulates emotions. Traumatic experiences are stored not only in our minds but also in our bodies in what's known as somatic memory. These experiences and how they live in our body after the event can lead to changes in how our body responds to stress, resulting in chronic alterations in our stress response system. This makes it more likely that we will be frozen in a stress response, always awaiting the next frightening or negative event, leading us to perceive even ordinary things as potential threats. This hypervigilance can keep us in a perpetual state of hyperarousal. Healing from trauma is possible, but it takes time and support. Trauma-informed therapies like somatic therapy and eye movement desensitization and reprocessing (EMDR) are effective in processing traumatic experiences. While healing won't erase the past, it can change how it affects our body today.

- **Generational trauma:** Even if you feel that you didn't experience trauma yourself, it's essential to recognize that unresolved trauma and stress within our family history can still affect us. Emerging evidence suggests that children can be affected by the trauma their parents or grandparents experienced before the children were even conceived. Mark Wolynn's book *It Didn't Start with You* explores how inherited family trauma shapes who we are, and how we can end the cycle. Many people continue to blame their parents for their problems, and while that may hold true, it's worth remembering that your parents had parents too, and *they* had parents too, and this goes way back. They were all just kids, learning from their parents. We are all doing the best we can with the tools and knowledge we have. We are all products of our familial and cultural backgrounds, yet we also have the ability as adults to be accountable for what *we can* *change* moving forward. A pattern of emotional conflict across generations may continue being passed down until someone is ready to resolve it. You can continue the cycle, or you can break it.

- **Life with ADHD:** If you lacked resources or support for your needs or weren't diagnosed with ADHD until later in life, you might have navigated through life by masking your struggles, pushing past your limits, and forcing yourself to fit in, all while hiding your challenges. Constant criticism and disappointment, from yourself and others around you, are typical for individuals with ADHD. This can lead your body to interpret everything as a threat, causing your nervous system to respond as if past events are occurring in the present. This ongoing stress and the internalized feelings of rejection or inadequacy can keep your body in a heightened state of stress and alertness. Additionally, you may have developed coping mechanisms such as overindulging in food, alcohol, or drugs to feel confident or to relax from the constant state of fight or flight, and these tactics might make you feel ashamed of or conflicted about using them, furthering the dysregulation.

Since all the systems in your body are connected, it's no surprise that a dysregulated nervous system can throw off the others as well. Constant stress triggers your body to release excess stress hormones like cortisol and adrenaline (also known as epinephrine), which can activate mast cells (a type of white blood cell) to release histamines. This leads to inflammation and immune system problems, including autoimmune diseases, in which the immune system mistakenly identifies the body's own tissues as threats.

A dysregulated nervous system can also impact gene expression through epigenetics, which occurs when environmental and lifestyle factors influence genes without actually changing them. Each cell in your body can turn genes on or off, and nervous system dysregulation can affect this process. For instance, having a gene linked to diabetes doesn't mean it's always active. In fact, two members of the same family could have the same diabetes gene. However, if one has a regulated nervous system and the other does not, the one with the dysregulated nervous system might be at a higher risk of activating the gene.

While it's tempting to shrug this off and think that that won't happen to you, it's crucial to recognize that the initial physical signs of nervous system dysregulation may be subtle. Symptoms like bloating, irritable bowel syndrome (IBS), shallow breathing, or signs of muscle tension such as neck pain or tight hips might seem random at first. However, when these issues persist over time, they could actually be red flags from the body. Ignoring these signals until we hit rock bottom or receive a diagnosis isn't uncommon. I tell you this to emphasize the importance of taking care of yourself, of noticing your nervous system; just because we can't see it doesn't mean it's not there. You take care of your nervous system, and it will take care of you.

---

*You take care of your nervous system,*
*and it will take care of you.*

---

Nervous system dysregulation can also lead to disconnection from yourself. You may feel out of touch with your emotions, bodily sensations, and sense of who you are. You may feel numb, empty, and overwhelmed, and have difficulty identifying and understanding the source of these feelings. You may not be aware of your body's needs, making it easy to neglect self-care and ignore signs of discomfort, hunger, and fatigue. You may find it challenging to define personal values, beliefs, and goals. You can feel disconnected from past experiences, present reality, and future vision, leading you to constantly question who you are and why you're here. It can be a struggle to define values and envision a positive future for yourself. When all of this gets to be too much, burnout hits. When we fall, we fall hard. And with the burnout come shame and fear. We feel weak for being frazzled, exhausted, and overwhelmed. For admitting that we need rest. For being more exhausted than other people our age who have it "harder."

## Reconnecting with Yourself

Living in this state of constant overwhelm takes a toll. Your body wasn't designed to be productive and give its all at all times, nor were you meant to force yourself to function at your peak under these conditions. In other words, we ADHD girls aren't resting and digesting enough, and we need to calm down. You might say, "No, I'm fine," because feeling this way is all you've ever known, but it's possible to shift your nervous system out of this dysregulated state and live a life where you're not always on edge, struggling to keep up with everything around you.

This life can't be attained with any fancy, state-of-the-art hacks. Through all the research I've done and by looking back on my personal experience, it's become clear to me that true health, happiness, and well-being aren't based on new, groundbreaking research that we haven't heard of before. A lot of what is being studied now and a lot of the advice out there recommend a return to ancient wisdom. You feel safe and hopeful when your body is able to flow with its ever-changing cycle of your hormones, when you can rest without guilt, when you let your eyes see sunshine instead of electronic screens first thing in the morning, when you eat real food, when you feel connected to your body and your heart, when you're able to move without pain and restriction, and when you find ways to complete the stress response cycle, engaging in activities that allow the body to return to a state of calm and safety. Many humans today are so out of touch with themselves that they don't remember (or maybe have never experienced) how it feels to feel truly alive with energy.

Throughout the rest of this chapter, I'll offer practices to help you regulate your nervous system by reconnecting with yourself. There is no one hack that will "heal" your dysregulated system overnight after suffering years of damage. Bringing your nervous system into balance is a journey that is unique to each person. Don't feel pressured to try every single one of the practices all at once. The point of giving you these options is to offer you the ability to choose what's the most helpful for your specific circumstances, even if it's something small. The daily moments, sacred practices, and little habits that connect you to yourself add up to create a healthy, happy life. And, hey—maybe what works today is different from what will work tomorrow. It depends on what season of life you're in. Pick and choose what works for you, whenever it works for you.

## BUILDING INTERNAL SAFETY

Our sense of safety refers to the feeling of security and well-being that we experience both internally and externally. Internally, it involves feeling secure within ourselves, trusting our instincts, emotions, and abilities. Externally, it involves feeling safe in our environment, whether it's our physical surroundings or our social interactions. This sense of safety is essential for emotional well-being and healthy relationships, because it allows us to navigate life with confidence and resilience.

You cannot fully experience health and happiness without it. This sensation comes when you acknowledge your authentic self, resulting in a feeling deep inside that it's safe to be you and that you can trust your own judgment and embrace who you are. This process might be difficult at times as you address past wounds along with the coping mechanisms you use to avoid feeling the pain, but as you foster a space of safety you gradually lighten these burdens. Establishing boundaries becomes easier because you realize that constantly prioritizing the feelings of others over your own only leads to internal turmoil. When you're smiling on the outside but dying on the inside, you've lost *your* own safety. You've lost connection with yourself.

Ultimately, internal safety nurtures a deeper sense of peace and fulfillment and empowers you to express yourself openly and honestly, enabling you to live life more fully and authentically. Keep this in mind—each suggestion I offer throughout this section is about sending little messengers to your nervous system to say, *Hey, we're safe here, we don't need to be on high alert. We can relax.*

## Put Your Basic Needs First

If you notice yourself in a state of fight or flight or are forced to stay in survival mode, it's time to show yourself that you are someone worthy of support, love, and care. This can start with listening to your body in the most basic way. For example, it can be as simple as going to the toilet when you need to pee instead of holding it in and promising you'll pee *after* you've completed the task at hand, thus putting the task first. Peeing when you need to might feel like a bit of an obvious and humiliating place to start, but if you don't do it when you're busting to go, how can you ever expect your nervous system to feel safe enough to relax and heal? You need to unlearn the habits that force you to ignore the most primal parts of yourself.

## Be Boring

One common way that ADHD sabotages our sense of safety is that it makes it easier for us to mistake routine and peace for boredom. This feeling of boredom leads us to crave the dopamine high of change. Impulsivity often wins the battle, leaving us with a wave of shame-filled regret and asking ourselves why we just did that. It's a cycle that many of us with ADHD are familiar with. We get comfy and calm with our day-to-day life, and we then create chaos out of the lack of stimulation.

As tempted as we are to give in to our impulses, especially in moments of emotional distress, we have to remember what our bodies actually need is moments of safety and peace. The irony here is that sometimes safety feels like the *furthest* thing from safe. When we're used to living in fight or flight, safety can feel unfamiliar or even scary. But just because we're used to a toxic cycle doesn't mean we don't have the option to choose something different. We *can* get comfortable with boredom, and thriving with ADHD requires us to do so. Boredom doesn't mean we're unhappy or out of alignment. After a lifetime of chaos and roller coasters, wouldn't it be nice just to complain about being bored, opting to pick up a book and read it instead of cutting our hair off or moving across the world again? Try it just this once. For a year. A month. A week. Imagine how soothing boredom might feel. Imagine watching the world go by. Taking a breath. Drinking some tea. Noticing the wind in the trees.

## Nurture Community Connection

One major reason why so many of us with ADHD experience nervous system dysregulation is because we're unable to see ourselves as connected to anything greater than ourselves. We might feel that we are in our own wee world, that we don't matter, that we aren't any good, that we are always misunderstood, and that we don't belong.

Despite this, we humans have an innate need for connection. **Slowing down and reconnecting with yourself is important, and in doing so you might notice a natural urge to connect with others, to be less isolated, to curate your own supportive community.** Not only is connection meeting an innate human need, but nervous system regulation can also happen *with* others.

When you're in a supportive community where you feel safe, accepted, and understood, you can start to coregulate with the people in this community. Coregulation happens when you're in the presence of a safe person who is more emotionally regulated than you are in that moment. (A person who is safe is someone whom you trust and feel comfortable with.) Your body experiences a sense of safety and relaxation, knowing that the people around you are witnessing your experiences and supporting them without judgment, allowing you to relax, drop into the moment, and be yourself without fear of criticism or harm.

For women in particular, social connection can be a way to react to stress. The "tend and befriend" theory proposed by psychologist Shelley E. Taylor suggests that we engage in nurturing behaviors ("tending") toward children or others in need of support and seek social support from others ("befriending") during times of stress. Our bodies also produce oxytocin, known as the love and bonding hormone. It is released not only through positive social interactions like touches or hugs, but also during times of stress to encourage bonding and connection (though chronic stress may suppress its levels because of the presence of other stress-related hormones such as cortisol and testosterone).

When I think about coregulation, I think about an early experience with my now fiancé, Ruairí. I was twenty-five, and we had just started seeing each other. We were starving after the gym so he made us food: a bowl with ground beef, rice, and veggies. As we were happily munching away, his cousin laughed and pointed out that we were both eating the same way. I hadn't even noticed that we had the same mannerisms when eating: fast, messy, and with spoons instead of forks. I remember feeling so different from the anxious girl I had been before. I felt relaxed with him. I knew he wouldn't judge me or be repulsed by me. I didn't always need to put my best foot forward.

This feeling of safety can also come from interactions with people outside your inner circle. Sharing your experiences with a therapist or coach who can offer you nonjudgmental support, understanding, and love can be deeply healing. Even people you don't interact with regularly can do the same. At the beginning of chapter 2, I asked you to imagine a woman who showed up late to a workout class and missed it. That woman was me. I had finally booked a workout class that I had been excited about trying for months, but I left for class with barely enough time to make it. It took just one commuting blip for me to end up missing the class.

Instead of letting this take away my chance to move, I wound up booking a last-minute yoga class instead. When I arrived, my teacher asked me how I was feeling and what I needed from the class. In the past, I would have been afraid to answer honestly. My brain has historically told me that admitting that I was anything other than absolutely fine was weak, embarrassing, and shameful.

But I told the truth. "I feel scattered, stressed, and overwhelmed." Closing my eyes, I said, "I need to feel calm and grounded." I let out a massive breath I'd been holding. Already, my body was showing me that sharing with my yoga teacher what was really going on had led to a moment of connection, which in turn had become a moment of healing. It turned out that that last-minute yoga class was exactly what I needed to settle my nervous system and bring me to a feeling of calm.

## COPING WITH REJECTION SENSITIVITY

Having a dysregulated nervous system can heighten emotional responses and amplify perceived threats, leaving many of us more sensitive to social rejection. Those of us with ADHD may face more of these social rejections than our non-ADHD peers, making the struggle even more real. Rejection sensitivity can lead to intense feelings of sadness, embarrassment, pain, and shame when we feel rejected or excluded. This hypersensitivity can stem from past experiences of rejection or trauma, which may have been what dysregulated the nervous system in the first place.

Sometimes we let the fear of not fitting in, of being teased, laughed at, or purposefully excluded, stop us from making new connections or even trying to engage with people at all. We might keep friends who aren't good for us or stay in unfulfilling relationships just to have *someone*, anyone! This, in turn, means we miss opportunities to coregulate with trusted people, which makes it even more challenging to self-soothe, regulate emotions effectively, and cope with rejection in a healthy manner.

It's inevitable that we will experience rejection, but if you find yourself screaming on the inside after blurting out something before thinking (Hi, ADHD) or feeling your heart sink when you realize you left a typo in before pressing "send" on an important email, I encourage you to return to the principles of self-compassion in chapter 2. Instead of thinking, *I'm so embarrassed*, remind yourself: *It happens! My intentions were pure. I was so excited that I didn't take a second to think.* No matter what your inner critic tries to tell you, remember that the other person isn't cringing half as much as you are. This embarrassment lives in your mind longer than in theirs, and you don't need to hold on to it. If they react badly, know that you'll meet many people who are wrong for you while you go about living your life. Not all of them will be lifelong partners and friends. The right people will love you for yourself.

Intense rejection sensitivity is not something you have to live with forever. As you regulate your nervous system and process unaddressed emotional wounds from the past, you'll notice your sensitivity to rejection slowly but surely decreasing.

## THE ART OF SLOWING DOWN

Contrary to popular belief, you do not have to fill every second of your day with doing something. You can just be. You can just rest. In fact, I would say that you *need* to just be and rest.

More than a decade ago, I was a fitness trainer with my own women-only gym. I did not know yet that I had ADHD, but looking back, I can see I was hyperfocused on my work. I was working many days from five in the morning until nine at night. I would spend my days at the gym doing a combination of one-on-one training sessions and boot-camp classes. After coming home at night, I'd eat a quick meal and stay up late into the night responding to messages from clients, only to wake up before dawn to head back to the gym. I adored every second of it. This was my calling. I felt like I was walking in my purpose. But I never stopped to take a break from that walk. I feared that if I slowed down, my success would all crumble away and I would be left with nothing.

I maxed myself out. I was drinking up to eight coffees a day just to keep up with it all. Many messages that I responded to took an emotional toll. They were often long, full of intense stories about trauma that I wasn't equipped to handle. I wanted to be there for my clients, but this meant I was always "on." After month after month of this, my body refused to keep going.

One morning, after waking up to my alarm to teach a 6:00 A.M. class, I stubbed my toe. I wobbled into the bathroom to brush my teeth and realized I'd forgotten to buy toothpaste. When I then dropped a glass of water on the floor, I broke into tears. Ru woke up to the noise. I had only thirty minutes before the class started. I sobbed, "I don't know what's wrong with me. I don't know why I'm crying, but I can't do it anymore. I can't go to work."

Ru, who was also a trainer at the time, covered for me

while I spent the entire morning sleeping. Feeling "tired" led to me taking a week off work, which led to me taking three weeks off work, which eventually led to me closing my gym full-stop and buying a one-way ticket to Dubai and working mostly online instead by turning my gym boot-camps into virtual boot-camps.

If we aren't careful, so many of us wait until the point of crisis to rest, giving burnout the opportunity to kill the things we love. Passion needs rest to nurture it. Don't fall for the "this time will be different" trap when you get going on an exciting new project. Make this time *actually* different by honoring your body and giving it the rest it desperately needs, even if your mind may not have consciously processed that you need it yet. Just as a kettle needs to be refilled before it can boil more water and make cups of tea, you too need to take the time to replenish yourself.

---

*Passion needs rest to nurture it.*

---

## Redefine Rest

Sleep might be the first thing that springs to mind when you think of rest, but it comes in different forms: physical, mental, social, creative, spiritual, sensory, and emotional. Rest can look like getting a massage, meditating, practicing deep breathing, enjoying someone's company, doodling, or painting.

The form of rest you need might look different from one day to the next, even from one moment to the next. Sometimes the solution to your tiredness is movement, especially when you spend too much time sitting. Playing tennis or going for a slow run might not seem like it will give your mind a break, but when your body experiences psychological stress, it naturally responds by anticipating movement. If we choose not to move and instead to remain sedentary, our internal stress can become trapped or stagnant. Sometimes your tiredness might stem from overstimulation from electronic screens. In this situation, spending time in nature without your phone or headphones might be exactly what you need.

**You can also think of rest as simply the art of slowing down.** No matter how your schedule looks, you can find a little moment to practice taking your time, even if it's for only twenty seconds. Take your morning cup of tea, for example. Don't just take that first sip mindlessly. *Bask* in it. Enjoy it. Be present with it. Notice the bubbles, the heat, the color. Feel the warm liquid touching your tongue. If you're used to running late and rushing around, see what it feels like to *just walk* for a block or two. Notice your body, feel your feet on the ground, put your hand over your heart, and just breathe; be *with* yourself.

## Say No and Let Go

As a society, we are hyperfixated on *doing* and praise others for how much they *do*. When people referred to me as the hardest worker in the room in the past, I would proudly wear what I perceived as praise like a badge of honor. Hard work comes naturally to women with ADHD when we're interested in what we're doing. Our brain's wiring allows us to easily hyperfocus on the things that interest us, and society's praise of that hyperfocus, specifically with regard to work, encourages us to maintain that level of intensity even when it no longer feels good.

We might even feel that we can't stop. The fear of falling behind can keep us working at an unsustainable pace, and we'll try to maintain this pace by working harder and faster, often at the expense of our health and sanity. Impulsivity has us agreeing to take on extra projects or commitments without fully considering the consequences, which we procrastinate on until the last minute. We have trouble coming up with ideas and tapping into our creativity because our mind is full of open loops. Unfinished projects, half-done tasks, and stress about what needs to get done leaves us with the impression that we're not doing enough. Because we've taken on so much, we don't even know where to start, and we sometimes end up doing nothing at all.

There are certain circumstances in which that "show up anyway" mentality is totally appropriate. Maybe you just had a baby. Maybe a loved one is sick. Maybe you're moving house. In these intense moments, many of us willingly opt in, knowing that life is going to be chaotic and out of balance for a little bit. But while there will be seasons of life where more output is required of you, it's not a way to live full-time. Not every moment in life is an extenuating circumstance. Not every opportunity is a matter of life or death. We need to learn when to accept and when to avoid the chaos and the imbalance.

How do you know when you need to say no? Trust your body. It will tell you when you're tired, need time to yourself, or simply don't feel like doing something. This message from your body might be a scream in the form of overwhelm. Feeling overwhelmed is one of the main signs that your nervous system is dysregulated; we feel a sense of powerlessness in our own bodies and lives. It's also one of the main signs that it's time to express yourself and say no.

There is no shame in saying no to the extra demands of work, society, or any other force that's weighing you down. Yes, it might feel embarrassing at first to ask for space or a break if you're not used to doing it. But it's okay to say no. It's okay to say not right now. "I'm too tired today," "I don't have the mental capacity right now," "I am overstimulated and need more space," "I feel overwhelmed so I can't commit," "I won't be there this time, but thanks for asking!," and "No, thanks!" are perfect responses to requests, invitations, and questions.

I know that saying no with confidence is a skill, but it is also a key that unlocks a life of peace, joy, and better self-esteem that I did not know was possible beforehand. On the other side of saying no, you'll see there are habits and systems of support available to you, making it so you don't need to suffer alone. I'll repeat that last part one time: You don't need to suffer alone. The world isn't continuing to spin because you're standing there panting for air, sweat dripping down your face, holding in your arms. Reach out to your people. Tell them you're exhausted, that you need a break. Let yourself be surprised by how much support you really have around you.

## MAKING WORK WORK FOR YOU

Your job or career takes up a massive part of your life, and it can be so easy to let its demands take over your life. Believe it or not, work doesn't *have* to make you miserable. It's so easy to get stuck in the trap of pushing yourself onward and comparing yourself to non-ADHD people who seem to be managing just fine. Maybe those people seem to be doing fine, but you don't know the whole story, you don't see behind the scenes. Maybe they take medication or maybe they have unhealthy coping strategies that they're not showing you.

To build a life where you can *just be* instead of a life where you're only *doing*, you might need to reassess whether your career, your job, and your working environment support you or are killing your spirit. Here are some questions whose answers can show you whether your work life is a source of dysregulation.

- Are moving and stimming allowed and encouraged? Or are you expected to stay seated at your desk until designated break times?

- Do you have access to quiet, dark, and empty rooms that you can use to decompress and regulate?

- Can you choose your work clothes or are you restricted to a certain type of fabric and a fit that cause sensory issues?

- Can you work remotely on some days of the week, and can this be at your discretion without giving advance notice?

- Are instructions, deadlines, and expectations for your work clearly outlined, or are they ambiguous?

On top of asking these questions, it's also worth trying to be mindful of what you need to work optimally and what you need from your colleagues. This might be as simple as asking for clarification about a project (and impressing your boss by showing how engaged you are with the task at hand), or it can look like asking for accommodations. ADHD is classified as a disability, and while this might feel hard to come to terms with, accepting the fact that you sometimes need extra help will, in turn, help you perform at your best and reduce any work-related stress. And if your job doesn't work with the wiring of your brain, I urge you to try to find flexible and remote career opportunities, if possible. Many people with ADHD also make great creatives, coaches, and entrepreneurs because of how their creative minds work. Your journey is the only one that matters, and if something is not working, it's okay to seek change.

## Dethrone Your Phone

We have grown so accustomed to the endless dopamine hits that come from our phones that the gadget has started to feel like an extension of ourselves. Even when it's nowhere near, I sometimes find my hand instinctively searching for it.

Many of us start our day by checking our email and various social media feeds on our phone. Whether or not you realize it, this practice exhausts you. Before your brain has had a chance to wake up properly, it already has to process the sudden, intense stream of stimulation coming from your social media scroll and absorb other people's noise, thoughts, and often negativity.

But the addiction to our phones goes beyond the dopamine hits we get from notifications and social media feeds. So many of us confuse being on our phones with being productive, but the truth is that pretending to work on your phone for the sake of productivity will only hinder you.

While our phones have made it easier than ever to get work done, to build and connect to a community, to find love, and to schedule a good workout, we need to set some boundaries.

- **Delete your social apps for one to two days a week:** Even better, if you can, delete the apps during the luteal phase, when you know your mood and energy are lower. In my experience, consuming other people's content can oftentimes be even more exhausting than creating it yourself. There's nothing worse than staring at TikTok and feeling like you should be posting or staying up-to-date with the accounts you follow, but not having the energy to do so.

- **Make your bedroom a phone-free zone:** Instead of relying on your phone to wake you up in the morning, get an alarm clock, ideally a sunrise clock. Before bed, turn off your phone and keep it in a separate room or on the other side of the bedroom so you have to get out of bed to switch it on. Use the settings on your phone to automatically lock yourself out of certain social media apps after 9:00 P.M.

- **Utilize a second, SIM-free phone or tablet:** I enjoy using my phone for guided practices like breathwork or Emotional Freedom Techniques (EFT tapping) in the morning and hypnosis at night. I keep an old SIM-free phone in my bedroom with only meditation, breathwork, and similar apps installed on it. I can't access emails, social media apps, or messages. As a result, I no longer have to rely on willpower to stop myself from scrolling while still in bed, because the apps simply aren't there. You could also program an iPad to work similarly.

- **Curate your feed:** As wild as it may sound, comparing yourself to others on social media is actually a form of stimulation seeking. You might notice yourself doing this when you feel bored and are scrolling social media for a dopamine hit. This comparison can trigger emotional reactions and provide a temporary boost in arousal, contributing to a sense of stimulation. Similarly, constantly seeking content that leaves you feeling angry and unhappy with the world is also a form of stimulation. Curate a healthier social media feed by identifying which accounts or types of content trigger feelings of envy, negativity, or hopelessness and unfollowing them. Look for a diverse range of accounts that uplift you and bring joy, such as those focused on nature, wellness, travel, or design. Find other people who share the same love for the hobbies you have and build healthy connections with them; instead of passively scrolling through their content, try actively supporting their journeys with a comment or message.

## Sleep

My old bedtime routine looked something like this: I would watch *Gilmore Girls* until 2:00 A.M., enjoy a quick scroll online, then collapse into bed at 2:30 A.M., when I finally felt exhausted enough to force myself to sleep. My partner, on the other hand, prefers to be asleep by 10:00 P.M. In the middle of a heated conversation about our incompatible nighttime routines, I heard myself say, "I have ADHD. I *can't* sleep as early as you."

If this sounds familiar, it's time to challenge this belief. Sleep is vital for our nervous system, especially if you have ADHD. Lack of good-quality sleep makes it harder to focus and to effectively store and retrieve positive memories, leading to a skewed, negative perception of our experiences. It makes us more sensitive emotionally, increasing mood swings and irritability. We're more likely to overreact to stressors and to feel on edge. Our brains have more trouble strengthening the connections between nerve cells and getting rid of toxins and waste.

I get that as someone with ADHD, it can be hard to get to bed. Our difficulty with self-regulation makes it tough to switch gears from daytime to bedtime routines, especially if we are hyperfocused on a stimulating activity such as binge-ing a TV series, playing video games, or falling down a social media scroll hole. We struggle to plan and take the steps needed to wind down, like brushing our teeth, changing into pajamas, and turning off screens. On some nights, it feels like there is so much to do, so we just sit in the comfort of the sofa for as long as we can until we collapse into bed.

To help ease the transition into bedtime, I've built what I like to think of as a little "sleep toolbox" of sorts that's full of strategies I use to help both my body and my mind wind down in the evenings. With the help of these tools, I'm happy to say that for the first time in years I have a consistent sleep schedule—usually falling asleep by 11:00 P.M. and waking up in the morning feeling refreshed. What follows are a few of my favorite strategies. There's a mix of low-effort and higher-effort practices here. I don't do each of these every night, but they have all made a difference. Feel free to adapt any of these as needed:

- **Stop eating three or four hours before bedtime:** Digestion can interfere with melatonin production. (This strategy is also the foundation for food timing; see page 205 to learn more.)

- **Go for a short walk after dinner:** Moving the body after your last meal of the day helps regulate blood sugar and triggers the release of endorphins, reducing stress and promoting relaxation.

- **Control your lighting:** Mimic the sun setting indoors by switching off all ceiling lights and only using softly lit lamps and lightbulbs that emit red light. If you find it hard to completely avoid screens at night, invest in a pair of blue-light-blocking glasses. Blocking blue light from electronics in the evening signals to the body that it's time to wind down and prepare for sleep and prevents it from interfering with the body's production of melatonin.

- **Take a magnesium glycinate supplement at least an hour before bed:** Magnesium glycinate can help you wind down, manage anxiety, and sleep better. (Learn more about how it works in the Supplements appendix on page 275.) You'll need to take magnesium glycinate specifically. Don't make the mistake I did and use magnesium citrate, which is used for constipation. To boost my magnesium intake further, I also draw a hot bath with Epsom salts and magnesium flakes and soak for twenty minutes to allow the magnesium to be absorbed through my skin. The bath promotes relaxation and soothes sore muscles, but because absorption of magnesium through the skin may be less efficient compared to oral supplementation, I don't skip my supplement.

- **Soothe yourself:** Play with some puzzles, work on a crossword, watch reruns of a comforting TV show, or read a book. If you choose to read, be mindful of avoiding books that might keep you awake. (I find that self-help and psychology books are usually too energizing and keep by my bed only books that help me relax, surrender, and switch off my thinking brain.) Avoid watching shows and movies that leave you on edge, such as true-crime documentaries. Accompany these activities with other little rituals such as sipping a hot cup of calming chamomile tea, placing a weighted blanket over your feet, or enjoying a heated neck pad to help you wind down and feel sleepy *before* you get into bed.

- **Create a sleep-friendly atmosphere:** Use a white-noise machine, an eye mask, a weighted blanket, or blackout curtains to block out noise and light disturbances that may disrupt sleep. Open your window for an hour before sleeping to make sure the room is cool, which will promote sleepiness. (You can close it before you fall asleep to avoid waking up freezing cold!)

- **Get light in your eyes:** Many sleep experts emphasize the significance of going to sleep before midnight, letting yourself be influenced by your body's response to changing light levels. Disrupted sleep patterns can interfere with this timing, resulting in lesser amounts of deep sleep overall. To maintain proper timing, aim for a consistent sleep and wake schedule. Getting morning sunlight in your eyes as soon as you wake up can also help you be sleepier that night, because natural light is a cue for circadian rhythms. So instead of trying to *force* yourself to sleep (which never works), get up earlier and get low-angle sunlight in your eyes the next day, while the sun is low in the sky after sunrise, to help reset your sleep schedule.

- **Try the 5 Things exercise**: While you're lying in bed, close your eyes. *Slowly* notice five things you can feel and five things you can hear, then open your eyes. With your eyes open, gently notice five things you can see. Repeat. Body scans like this trigger the body's relaxation response, which lowers the cortisol level and reduces muscle tension. By connecting to sensations in the body, you become more grounded in the present and less attached to the racing thoughts or worries keeping you stimulated and awake. This body scan is a key part of my nighttime routine, and I also use it if I feel an anxiety attack coming on or start to disassociate.

- **Listen to hypnosis**: Sleep hypnosis audio can be a great tool in helping you fall asleep. It involves listening to someone guiding you into relaxation and drawing you into a trancelike state using words, storytelling, and visual cues. The tool may increase the amount of time you spend in deep sleep, which is necessary for both memory and healing. Hypnosis can reprogram negative thought patterns and beliefs about sleep and facilitate a smoother transition into sleepiness and overall a better relationship with sleep. As someone with ADHD, you might find hypnosis and hypnotherapy quite effective and enjoyable because you are naturally able to slip into an imaginative trancelike state.

## YOUR OPTIMAL BEDTIME

It's not just about *how much* sleep we get, but the *quality* of that sleep. The best way to maximize the quality of sleep is to go to sleep at the right time and in alignment with our circadian rhythms. For many people, melatonin naturally rises within a specific window of time each night. (For most people, this happens between 10:00 P.M. and midnight, though it might be earlier or later, depending on your individual circadian rhythm.) A restorative form of deep sleep takes place within those first few hours of sleep. During this time, the glymphatic system clears waste from the brain, a process that helps protect us from neurodegenerative diseases. Growth hormones that support neuroplasticity—

the brain's ability to adapt and change—are released. This type of sleep also boosts the health of the prefrontal cortex, the part of our brain associated with executive function, including our ability to plan, organize, and prioritize. Going to bed during the window when our melatonin level peaks ensures that we can fall asleep deeply enough to enjoy these benefits.

## GET OUT OF YOUR HEAD AND INTO YOUR BODY

In this section, you'll find a variety of practices designed to further promote nervous system regulation. From somatic shaking to humming, these exercises all help promote relaxation, reduce the production of stress hormones, improve circulation, facilitate movement out of stuck responses, and aid in processing and regulating emotions. By engaging in these exercises, you are acknowledging the importance of your body in emotional regulation. Rather than analyze feelings intellectually, these exercises can provide a direct pathway to engage with bodily sensations, go beyond just words, and work with the body.

Now that we've discussed the *why,* let's dive into the *what.* Without further ado, check out some of my favorite practices for regulating the nervous system, all of which can be turned into rituals to weave into your everyday life.

## Somatic Shaking

You know how animals shake themselves off after getting into a stressful tizzy and then just go back to what they were doing as if nothing has happened? We humans are meant to do the same. Somatic shaking sounds fancy, but all it describes is the act of shaking out your body to release stress and fear and deactivate your sympathetic nervous system. Every night before bed, I discharge the stress of the day by shaking each of my limbs. Because it can be quite activating and keep you awake, I practice it slowly and gently.*

## Mindful Movements

There are many activities, such as reformer Pilates, gymnastics, tennis, and boxing, that require you to be present with your body and focus on your next move. I find my mind wanders when I'm in the gym lifting weights, but when I'm in a class where I need to try to balance on one leg or hit a ball,

---

* You can delve deeper into somatic therapies by finding a provider trained in trauma therapy. Specifically, TRE®, or Tension and Trauma Releasing Exercises, is a somatic body-based practice for people coping with stress, anxiety, trauma, or PTSD. It's a great option for addressing the traumatic experiences that have become stuck in our bodies. Because you'll be working on releasing deep muscular patterns of stress, tension, and trauma through neurogenic tremors, I recommend completing this work with a practitioner there to tend to you. I have Ruairí to thank for introducing me to TRE and guiding me through it.

I'm more likely to remain engaged with what I'm doing in the moment. Practices that combine gentle movement with breathwork, such as yoga and qigong, can also foster mindfulness, as well as induce relaxation, enhance flexibility, and heighten your body awareness. Yin yoga, which involves holding poses for three to five minutes, is especially helpful for activating the parasympathetic nervous system because of its slow-paced nature.

## Free-Form Movements

Movements that don't come with any rules, such as dancing, can be powerful tools for emotional expression. When done without the worry of the judgment of others or yourself, these movements can help your body release shame and tension. Simply dancing along to a high-vibe song while making your breakfast alone is a powerful way to connect with your body as you start your day.

Free-form movements are especially helpful if you're experiencing a panic attack or intense anxiety because they help you complete a stress response. If you're feeling activated, your brain might seem hell-bent on convincing you that there is danger and you might feel an urge to hide from this imaginary "danger." Resist that urge. Get on the floor and let your body move it out instead. Yes, rolling around on the floor will help. Move in a way that feels intuitive. There's no right or wrong way.

## Lymphatic Drainage and Fascia Release

The fascia is a connective tissue that surrounds your muscles and organs. It also absorbs and carries stress from physical and emotional trauma. When trauma is stored in the fascia, it can lead to hypervigilance and chronic pain and make you more likely to stay stuck in fight-or-flight mode or experience emotional dysregulation.

The lymphatic system, located within the fascia, removes waste excreted from cells, prevents toxin buildup, and transports immune cells. When stored trauma compresses the fascia and causes knots to form, the lymphatic river becomes blocked. This is problematic because the blockage can lead to toxin buildup, causing inflammation and health issues. It also impedes nutrient and oxygen delivery to cells and hinders immune cell movement, making it harder to fight infections. Practices like myofascial release, massage, stretching, and lymphatic drainage movements can relieve tension in your fascia and improve lymphatic flow.

Massage and mobility work, such as myofascial release, treat fascia knots by breaking up adhesions and releasing tension. These practices can be performed at home on your own using tools like foam rollers and massage balls, or by seeing a myofascial release practitioner for more precise treatment. You can practice self-massage around the collarbones to open up the lymph nodes, promoting drainage and reducing blockages. Trampolining is also effective for improving lymphatic flow. The gentle bouncing helps open and close the lymphatic valves, encouraging the flow of lymph fluid throughout the body. Using a mini trampoline for a few minutes each day, especially in the morning, can be a beneficial part of your self-care routine.

## Experience Nature

What makes time spent in nature healing for our nervous system is not just noticing it, but actively *engaging* with it using our senses. Instead of watching birds fly by or snapping photos, immerse yourself in nature by sitting under a tree and feeling its shade or walking barefoot on the grass. Touch and smell plants to experience their textures and scents, swim in the ocean, or garden with your bare hands. Being in natural environments has been found to reduce sympathetic nervous system activity, bring on a state of relaxation, reduce blood pressure, and promote healthier nervous system function. Exposure to natural light helps regulate your circadian rhythms and your production of neurotransmitters that help manage things like your mood, sleep, and stress level. When we ground ourselves in the present moment and focus on sensory experiences such as sight, sound, touch, taste, and smell, we redirect our attention away from worries and stressors, bringing a greater sense of connection to our bodies and surroundings. This process helps to calm the nervous system by reducing the activation of the stress response and promoting a state of relaxation.

## Hum

Take a breath and then hum on the exhale. Humming puts your parasympathetic nervous system back in charge by stimulating your vagus nerves and triggering the release of acetylcholine and GABA, neurotransmitters that promote a sense of calm and reduce your stress level.[*] If you attend yoga classes, you might have been asked to hum at the end of a class. Join in the next time to soothe your nervous system. Don't be shy!

## Bilateral Stimulation

Bilateral stimulation involves stimulating both sides of the body simultaneously, typically with alternating taps, sounds,

* Loud gargling with water and singing also have the same effect. It turns out there's a reason why singing in the shower feels so good!

or eye movements, which activate both sides of the brain and help you move out of a stress response. There are many different ways to relax with bilateral stimulation.[*]

Here's one of my favorite options:

1. Hold one of your arms straight out in front of you. Move it to the right and let your eyes follow it without moving your head.

2. Once your arm has reached as far to the right as it can go, let your head follow until it's aligned with your hand again.

3. Move that arm back to your center starting point with only your eyes following. Once your arm is in the middle again, follow it with your head.

4. Repeat steps 1 through 3, but move your arm to the left. Alternate sides for as long as you need to. If you yawn or sigh deeply, it's a sign you're calming down and moving into a relaxed state.

---

[*] Bilateral stimulation is also a therapeutic technique commonly utilized in eye movement desensitization and reprocessing (EMDR) therapy, a well-established method for treating trauma. When administered by a trained practitioner, bilateral stimulation has been shown to be effective in addressing trauma-related symptoms and facilitating emotional healing. Early research is also indicating it's effective in helping with ADHD challenges.

## Meditation

Meditation allows you to enter a state of deep relaxation, giving your nervous system a real opportunity to decompress. Regular meditation can enhance neuroplasticity, helping your brain restructure itself and create new neural connections. When your brain can reorganize and form new connections easily, it improves how well you can think, regulate your emotions, and create new, healthy habits. You'll be better equipped to handle stress and cultivate more patience.

If you have ADHD, you might have found meditation boring in the past. I recommend starting with more active forms of meditation, such as guided meditations that you can listen to rather than silent ones. Sounds and words that bring you calm and remind you that you're exactly where you're meant to be—and on the path toward becoming the future self you dream of—will help motivate you to go to the gym, eat a nourishing meal, and start choosing peace over chaos in everyday moments. Simply noticing where you are is a form of meditation; by bringing your complete attention to your surroundings—feeling the grass beneath your feet, noticing the sounds of the birds, and being fully present—you are practicing mindfulness meditation.

## *Breathe*

In *Breath: The New Science of a Lost Art,* author James Nestor explores how modern humans have deviated from proper breathing patterns, often by breathing too quickly and shallowly. Improper breathing can negatively impact brain and nervous system functioning by keeping our bodies in a constant fight-or-flight response. Fast and shallow breaths signal to our brains that there is something to be stressed about, making it harder to come back to a healthy baseline after stressful moments.

Breathwork, exercises designed to help us regulate our breathing, can calm the nervous system. Just a few minutes of correct breathing every day tells your nervous system it can relax.

When I'm stressed, my favorite breathwork technique is to simply *extend my exhale.* I'll breathe in for a count of four and then blow out for eight for a few breaths. Exhaling for a longer duration than inhaling allows the body to expel more carbon dioxide, which helps maintain the proper balance of oxygen and carbon dioxide in the bloodstream. When I'm struggling with a hyperactive brain that won't let me sleep, I love to practice box breathing using the image of a pod on a Ferris wheel.

1. Breathe in slowly for a count of four seconds, feeling your lower abdomen fill up. In your mind, imagine the pod on the Ferris wheel going up.

2. Pause at the top for four seconds, holding your breath and imagining that the Ferris wheel has stopped.

3. Slowly exhale through your mouth for four seconds, letting your abdomen deflate toward your spine, similar to how the Ferris wheel pod comes down and around.

4. Hold your breath for four seconds at the bottom, imagining that the Ferris wheel pod has reached the ground.

5. Repeat these steps as needed to calm your mind and body.

## Play

Play is a fundamental part of well-being, but somewhere between childhood and adulthood we stop doing it. Play puts us in a state of flow and encourages self-expression, creativity, and spontaneity. Play is the biochemical and neurological opposite of trauma in the body. Unlike trauma, which can trigger stress responses and negative physiological effects, play is voluntary and intrinsically motivated. Play is important for nervous system regulation because it offers a natural way to engage the parasympathetic nervous system to help the body relax and recover from stress, shifting the nervous system out of stuck stress responses such as hyperarousal or hypoarousal. How did you play when you were younger, before you had access to phones, screens, and video games? Bring some of that joy, fun, and ease back into your life. Maybe revisit childhood hobbies or interests, like collecting, crafting, or dancing. Or enhance your living space with more games and fun activities. For instance, I have a ping-pong set that holds a permanent spot on the kitchen table. Playing a game gives me endless laughs and taps into my playful and mischievous side. It's even more helpful if I'm feeling moody.

Play is not limited to physical activities; it can also include mental activities like puzzles, crosswords, anagrams, and board games. These games help with problem-solving, learning new words, and recognizing patterns, which encourages mental flexibility and trains the brain to strengthen executive function and memory. You can also cultivate playfulness within yourself by embracing spontaneity, adventure, and lightheartedness, allowing yourself to be fully present in the moment and laughing freely without worrying about the outcome. By nurturing a playful mindset, you can bring more joy, creativity, and vitality into your everyday experiences.

## Process Uncomfortable Emotions

Many of us have difficulty expressing uncomfortable emotions, especially anger. And who can blame us? As women, we have been told by society for centuries that we are supposed to be agreeable, pleasant, and selfless—there's no room for anger in the role our culture has laid out for us. These patterns start for many of us at an early age. When you don't have your basic emotional needs met in early life, the nervous system creates coping patterns like "people pleasing" or "being a good girl" as a means of seeking that approval, acceptance, or love. This might also involve suppressing feelings of anger or other emotions to maintain harmony. Over time you get used to the praise that comes with acting this way, reinforcing the pattern. But bottling our true feelings is extremely costly to our health. In an article for *TIME*, psychologist and host of the podcast *Heal with It* Maytal Eyal, PhD, writes, "It seems that the very virtues our culture rewards in women—agreeability, extreme selflessness, and suppression of anger—may predispose us to chronic illness and disease." In his book *The Myth of Normal*, Gabor Maté, MD, draws a correlation between repressed emotions and autoimmune disease, a condition associated with nervous system dysregulation. "Hyperfunctioning on top of hidden distress is a recurring theme among the many autoimmune patients I've encountered," he writes.

Feeling anger is our body's signal that something isn't right—it can indicate that we're being harmed or that our needs aren't being fulfilled. When channeled appropriately, it is a boundary-setting energy meant to be expressed outward. But when we don't feel it is safe to express our anger, it instead goes inward. In other words, the fight-or-flight stress response that gets triggered when we first feel the anger rise within us goes unfinished, leaving it looping inside us and throwing our nervous system off-balance. Now, I'm not suggesting you get violent or start screaming at the innocent pedestrian who bumped into you on the street. As Dr. Maté writes in his book *When the Body Says No,* "Anger does not require hostile acting out." The key is to not suppress the experience of anger. Chronic repression of anger can escalate into a pattern of aggressive behavior over time, causing overreactions to everyday situations and leading to feelings of irritability, annoyance, or even rage. Refusing to address the root cause of your anger can also leave you channeling it into the wrong places, impulsively lashing out and harboring hostility.

Rather than pushing your anger down, allow yourself to feel angry instead. Observe and experience your emotions without judging them or trying to resist them. Anger is a natural emotion; there's no need to feel ashamed or consider it wrong. Before you talk about it with someone you trust or write about it in a journal, practice moving it out first. **Your nerves activate your muscles to contract when angry. This means that your** body wants to move into action, so let it. **This movement is what will help process the emotion. Try stomping your feet as you would have when you were a child. Or try one of my favorite movements: Lie on the floor, squeeze your knees into your chest as tightly as you can, then relax. Repeat this a few times.** Let the feelings flow naturally and then journal about it or talk to someone. Releasing built-up emotions and addressing past challenges can help regulate the nervous system by finally allowing that trapped tension stored in the body to be discharged and promote the body's innate healing mechanisms. By facing these emotions instead of suppressing them, you open the door to true healing.*

Q: Learning about these practices has only made me feel more overwhelmed. What if I don't remember to—or can't—do all these things?

A: The hard truth about adapting to new ways of living is that the process of learning is messy, and patterns are sometimes hard to change. You probably *will* forget one or another of these practices at some point. You probably *will* experience overwhelm and burnout again.

* To dive deeper into this work, I recommend checking out the work of Peter A. Levine, PhD. He holds doctorates in both medical biophysics and psychology and has spent fifty years studying and treating stress and trauma. He created Somatic Experiencing® (SE™), which aims to resolve symptoms of stress, shock, and trauma that accumulate in our bodies and nervous systems.

I speak from personal experience. Thanks to the work I was doing to regulate my nervous system and de-stress, I was starting to inch out of survival mode. But despite my best efforts, I still wasn't resting enough. I would finish a session of somatic trauma therapy, dive straight into responding to work messages, and work late into the night.

Burnout eventually came for me again. It wasn't until I experienced a terrible bout of food poisoning that I realized how hard I had been pushing myself. After spending a night vomiting, all I could do the next day was lie on my sofa and stare at the ceiling. I thought, *How the fuck did I get here? How burned out am I that this feels like such magic?*

I tell you this story because sometimes in life we can repeat a pattern over and over and over again without learning from it until, of course, we finally do. Be patient with yourself. You'll get there. Instead of worrying you're doing it wrong or that there's too much to remember, allow curiosity to take over and trust that the small steps you're taking to show your nervous system that it can relax will add up. The tiniest actions can send a message of safety: humming your favorite song, listening to the birds sing, having a little dance, softening your shoulders and unclenching your jaw, allowing your exhale to be longer than your inhale, letting your eyes slowly wander the room, and noticing the feeling of your spine against your chair.

# Appendix: Supplements

I've always enjoyed experimenting with different supplements to help optimize my health, but last year when I was struggling badly with PMDD, I started considering their benefits more seriously. Here, I share the supplements, beyond the most commonly taken ones and your average multivitamin, that have given me the best benefits.

Some supplements might contain adaptogens, and I like to practice supplement cycling if I'm taking one of them. Adaptogens, such as ashwagandha, rhodiola, ginseng, maca, and reishi, are herbal medicines used for stress support to help the body return to its normal physiological function. Supplement cycling means if I start an adaptogen supplement for stress support, I'll use it for a few weeks or months and then stop using it or swap to a supplement without the adaptogen. I recommend taking breaks from these supplements to prevent tolerance from developing and for the adaptogen to maintain its effectiveness on the body and to minimize potential side effects.

When shopping for supplements, try to avoid ones containing artificial dyes and sweeteners. So many of us take these supplements thinking we're doing something good for our bodies when in reality we're ingesting ingredients that may make our ADHD symptoms worse.

Finally, it's essential to do your own research and also consult with your healthcare provider before starting any new supplement regimen, especially with adaptogens, to ensure that they are suitable for your individual needs and health status, especially if you have any health conditions, are taking other medications, are pregnant, or are trying to conceive.

MAGNESIUM GLYCINATE: Magnesium is an essential mineral for the entire body, especially the brain. It is the fourth-most-abundant mineral in the body and is involved in more than three hundred biochemical processes. Many of us have a magnesium deficiency because modern agricultural practices have depleted nutrients from our soil. Factors like water filtration, processed foods, stress, and medications further contribute. There are different types of magnesium, and while taking a magnesium blend is great, you'll specifically want to look for **magnesium glycinate** if you're dealing with anxiety and poor sleep. Magnesium glycinate helps control how the body reacts to stress by working with the hypothalamic-pituitary-adrenal (HPA) axis and by helping to increase the activity of GABA, a neurotransmitter known for its calming effects on the brain, promoting relaxation and better sleep. Research suggests that those of us with ADHD may have lower GABA levels or impaired GABA receptor function compared to those without it, which could contribute to the anxiety, racing thoughts, and impulsivity often present in ADHD. Finally, magnesium plays a role in vitamin D absorption because our bodies can't properly use vitamin D without a sufficient magnesium level.

**METHYLATED B VITAMINS:** You may be spending money on B vitamins that your body can't use. Some B vitamins, like vitamin $B_9$ (folic acid) and vitamin $B_{12}$, need an enzyme we produce called MTHFR to become active and useful in the body. This enzyme helps them make and repair DNA, as well as produce neurotransmitters. The methylated form of **vitamin $B_9$** is called methylfolate (make sure the supplement lists methylfolate, or folate, as an ingredient instead of folic acid). The methylated form of **vitamin $B_{12}$** is called methylcobalamin (make sure the supplement lists that as an ingredient instead of vitamin $B_{12}$, cyanocobalamin, or hydroxocobalamin).

If your MTHFR gene has mutations, it can mess up this process and affect how your body processes nutrients, which can impact brain function and potentially increase the risk of a range of conditions like anemia, depression, anxiety, and miscarriage. Mutations in MTHFR have been linked to more than sixty conditions, including ADHD, which might mean you could have low folate levels. Not having enough of these vitamins may affect how the brain and hormones communicate. By some estimates, up to 40 percent of the population may have an MTHFR mutation of some kind. Having an MTHFR variant doesn't always mean that you need medical treatment; it could just mean that you need to take a methylated vitamin B supplement. If you're curious to discover your individual MTHFR status, many at-home genetic testing kits offer screening for MTHFR.

OMEGA-3 FATS: Omega-3 fats play a key role in brain health, neurotransmitter function, and communication between your brain and your hormones. They also reduce inflammation. (You can refer back to "Eat Fats," page 203, in chapter 7, for more information.) Remember to read the ingredients of the omega-3 fat supplements you're taking. There's a chance you may be taking a supplement with a blend of omega-3s, -6s, and -9s. While getting a balance of the three is important, adding more omega-6s when you already have too much (thanks to modern-day diets) isn't helpful.

SAFFRON: Saffron contains antioxidants and anti-inflammatory compounds that protect the brain from stress and inflammation. Saffron regulates mood-related neurotransmitters like serotonin and dopamine and may affect cortisol levels. In a study comparing saffron to fluoxetine (Prozac) for treating PMDD, thirty milligrams of saffron daily was found to reduce PMDD symptoms in the same way as Prozac, but without the side effects. A study done on adolescents with ADHD found saffron to be similarly effective as methylphenidate, a type of ADHD medication, for hyperactivity. Saffron's neuroprotective properties and antioxidant effects help alleviate ADHD symptoms by improving attention, reducing impulsivity, and regulating mood. Its use during pregnancy is generally not recommended.

VITAMINS $D_3$ WITH $K_2$: Vitamin $D_3$, also known as cholecalciferol, is the preferred form of vitamin D for supplementation because it more effectively raises blood levels of vitamin D compared to other forms like vitamin $D_2$. Additionally, vitamin $D_3$ is the form naturally produced by the body when skin is exposed to sunlight, so it is more biologically active. Adequate levels of vitamin D are crucial for mood and hormonal balance. A low level of vitamin D can make you feel low, even depressed, especially during the darker months of the year and if you live with seasonal affective disorder (SAD).

Studies have found that children with ADHD have lower vitamin D levels than healthy controls, and that low maternal vitamin D levels during pregnancy increase the likelihood of a child being diagnosed with ADHD. Vitamin $K_2$ is essential for proper vitamin D absorption and utilization in the body. Many vitamin D supplements have added $K_2$ for this reason.

VITEX AGNUS-CASTUS FRUIT: *Vitex agnus-castus* fruit, also known as vitex or chasteberry, is a plant commonly used to support hormonal balance in women. It's often recommended for PMS and PMDD, and some women use it to regulate their progesterone production after stopping hormonal birth control. *Vitex agnus-castus* primarily affects the hypothalamic-pituitary-gonadal (HPG) axis, which regulates reproductive hormone production, including estrogen, progesterone, testosterone, and luteinizing hormone, which are essential for menstrual cycle regulation and fertility. It has also been shown to stimulate dopamine receptors in the brain, helping to reduce mood-related symptoms associated with depression, PMS, and PMDD. I take capsules that also have added milk thistle, which is great for liver health. (A tired, overburdened liver can't effectively detoxify excess hormones, causing hormonal imbalances.) *Vitex agnus-castus* fruit use during pregnancy or breastfeeding is not recommended.

# Acknowledgments

I couldn't have written this book without the amazing support of so many wonderful people.

First off, a special thank-you to my partner, Ruairí Stewart, who has been by my side for the last ten years. Your unwavering support, love, and understanding have carried me through the toughest times and the greatest moments. I love you.

I have another massive thank-you for the incredible team at my agency, Dystel, Goderich & Bourret, especially Michael Bourret and Amy Bishop-Wycisk. I appreciate your support and dedication to this project.

To my fantastic team at Rodale Books, you've been a dream to work with. A special shout-out to my editor, Elysia Liang. Your insights and edits have truly helped me shape this book into something special. I'm so grateful for your wisdom, patience, and encouragement. Thank you for teaching me how to write a book. A heartfelt thank-you to Candice Jalili for the endless WhatsApp messages and the long voice notes that we sent back and forth. Your support helped me stay focused throughout, especially on those deadlines.

And to Danielle Curtis, what can I say? Thank you for that unexpected email on a random Tuesday afternoon, asking me to write this book. Your faith in me has been truly life-changing.

To my family and friends who have always encouraged my dreams, your love and support mean the world to me.

To my clients and the women I've shared meaningful conversations with over the years, thank you for trusting me and allowing me to be a part of your journey. Your experiences and stories have been a huge source of inspiration, contributing immensely to the creation of this book.

Thank you to the countless mentors, teachers, guides, therapists, and healers I've worked with over the years. Your experience and guidance have shaped me in more ways than I can express.

Above all, I want to give glory to God for guiding me through this journey and blessing me with the strength and inspiration to complete this book. Writing a book is a lifelong dream come true, and I count my lucky stars every day.

*To all of you,* thank you for being here. I wish health and happiness to you all.

# Notes

## Chapter 1: Change How You See ADHD

9 **boys are almost twice as likely:** "Data and Statistics on ADHD," Centers for Disease Control and Prevention, May 16, 2024, www.cdc.gov /adhd/data/index.html?.

16 **Building new habits:** Grace Weintrob, "How to Rewire Your Brain," Columbine Health Systems Center for Healthy Aging, Colorado State University, May 31, 2022, www.research.colostate.edu/healthyagingcenter /2022/05/31/how-to-rewire-your-brain.

18 **One study published in the *European Journal of Social Psychology*:** Phillippa Lally, Cornelia H. M. van Jaarsveld, Henry W. W. Potts, and Jane Wardle, "How Are Habits Formed: Modelling Habit Formation in the Real World," *European Journal of Social Psychology* 40, no. 6 (July 16, 2009): 998–1009, doi.org/10.1002/ejsp.674.

31 **factors such as stress, poor diet:** Kelly Ryan, "Five Ways Junk Food Changes Your Brain," RMIT University, September 19, 2016, www.rmit .edu.au/news/all-news/2016/sep/five-ways-junk-food-changes-your-brain; Michael A. P. Bloomfield, Robert A. McCutcheon, Matthew Kempton, Tom P. Freeman, and Oliver Howes, "The Effects of Psychosocial Stress on Dopaminergic Function and the Acute Stress Response," *eLife* 8 (November 12, 2019), doi.org/10.7554/elife.46797.

## Chapter 2: Practice Self-Compassion

39 **"Don't believe":** Steven Bartlett, "The ADHD Doctor: 'I've Scanned 250,000 Brains' You (Steven Bartlett) Have ADHD! & Coffee Is Damaging Your Brain!!! Dr Daniel Amen," *The Diary of a CEO with Steven*

*Bartlett* [podcast], October 2023, 60:50, open.spotify.com/episode/79xII
5djWfXn0FO67OPUFG?si=I8y0APOYR4OwpsBkUsOvkA.

## Chapter 3: Change How You See Yourself

63  **activates our body's stress responses:** Helena Boschi, "The Neuro-
science of Change: Why Changing Course Is Painful for the Brain,"
Welldoing.org, September 24, 2020, welldoing.org/article/the
-neuroscience-change-why-changing-course-painful-for-brain.

63  **generational trauma passed down:** Stephen G. Matthews and David I.
Phillips, "Transgenerational Inheritance of Stress Pathology," *Experimen-
tal Neurology* 233, no. 1 (January 2012): 95–101, doi.org/10.1016
/j.expneurol.2011.01.009.

70  **visualizing having done something:** Catherine Brandon,
"Visualisation—It's Like Weight-Lifting for the Brain," Springer Nature
Research Communities, November 1, 2020, communities.springernature
.com/posts/visualisation-it-s-like-weight-lifting-for-the-brain.

71  **When you think about your future self:** Hal Hershfield, "How Can We
Help Our Future Selves?," TEDxEast, posted September 9, 2014, TEDx
Talks, YouTube video, 11:56, www.youtube.com/watch?v=tJotBbd7MwQ.

92  **listening to music can modulate:** Luisa Speranza, Salvatore Pulcrano,
Carla Perrone-Capano, Umberto di Porzio, and Floriana Volpicelli,
"Music Affects Functional Brain Connectivity and Is Effective in the
Treatment of Neurological Disorders," *Reviews in the Neurosciences* 33,
no. 7 (March 24, 2022): 789–801, pubmed.ncbi.nlm.nih.gov/35325516.

## Chapter 4: Move More

97  **increasing dopamine and norepinephrine levels in the brain:**
"6 Things to Know About Adderall," Lee Health, last updated February 3,
2021, www.leehealth.org/health-and-wellness/healthy-news-blog
/top-trends/6-things-to-know-about-adderall.

97  **You know what else increases:** "Regular Exercise Benefits Both Mind
and Body: A Psychiatrist Explains," Mid-Atlantic Permanente Medical
Group, December 22, 2021, mydoctor.kaiserpermanente.org/mas/news
/regular-exercise-benefits-both-mind-and-body-a-psychiatrist-explains
-1903986.

99  **Exercise increases blood flow to the brain:** Jordan S. Querido and
A. William Sheel, "Regulation of Cerebral Blood Flow During Exercise,"
*Sports Medicine* 37, no. 9 (January 1, 2007): 765–82, pubmed.ncbi.nlm
.nih.gov/17722948.

100  **the brain has the ability to generate:** Chen Wang, Zhen Qian, and Jun-
jun Ding, "The Generation of New Neurons in the Adult Brain," *Nature
Medicine* 25 (2019): 1227–35, doi.org/10.1038/s41591-019-0375-9.

100  **triggers the release of feel-good neurotransmitters:** "Working Out

Boosts Brain Health," American Psychological Association, March 4, 2020, www.apa.org/topics/exercise-fitness/stress.

101 **protection against dopamine depletion:** Kelly McGonigal, "Five Surprising Ways Exercise Changes Your Brain," *Greater Good,* UC Berkeley, January 6, 2020, greatergood.berkeley.edu/article/item/five_surprising _ways_exercise_changes_your_brain.

108 **When studying the Blue Zones:** Dan Buettner, *The Blue Zones: 9 Lessons for Living Longer from the People Who've Lived the Longest* (Washington, DC: National Geographic, 2012).

109 **the people who live the longest:** Board on Population Health and Public Health Practice, "Lessons from the Blue Zones®," in *Business Engagement in Building Healthy Communities: Workshop Summary* (Washington, DC: National Academies Press, 2015), www.ncbi.nlm .nih.gov/books/NBK298903.

114 **provide a workout for the brain:** "These 5 Physical Activities Improve Brain Health," Amen Clinics, November 2, 2021, www.amenclinics.com /blog/these-5-physical-activities-improve-brain-health.

115 **those who played tennis:** Peter Schnohr, James H. O'Keefe, Andreas Holtermann, Carl J. Lavie, Peter Lange, Gorm Boje Jensen, and Jacob Louis Marott, "Various Leisure-Time Physical Activities Associated with Widely Divergent Life Expectancies: The Copenhagen City Heart Study," *Mayo Clinic Proceedings* 93, no. 12 (September 4, 2018): 1775–85, www.mayoclinicproceedings.org/article/S0025-6196(18)30538 -X/fulltext.

### Chapter 5: Add More Protein

138 **incorporating protein into our diets:** Berrak Basturk, Zeynep Koc Ozerson, and Aysun Yuksel, "Evaluation of the Effect of Macronutrients Combination on Blood Sugar Levels in Healthy Individuals," *Iran Journal of Public Health* 50, no. 2 (February 9, 2021): 280–87, doi.org/10.18502 /ijph.v50i2.5340.

138 **Multiple studies have shown that people:** Lucy Riglin, Beate Leppert, Christina Dardani, Ajay K. Thapar, Frances Rice, Michael C. O'Donovan, George Davey Smith, et al., "ADHD and Depression: Investigating a Causal Explanation," *Psychological Medicine* 51, no. 11 (August 2021): 1890–97, www.ncbi.nlm.nih.gov/pmc/articles/PMC8381237.

139 **A 2020 paper found that people who ate:** Yan Li, Caixia Zhang, Suyun Li, and Dongfeng Zhang, "Association Between Dietary Protein Intake and the Risk of Depressive Symptoms in Adults," *British Journal of Nutrition* 123, no. 11 (February 20, 2020): 1290–301, doi.org/10.1017 /s0007114520000562.

142 **More than half of women with PCOS:** "Diabetes and Polycystic Ovary Syndrome (PCOS)," Centers for Disease Control and Prevention,

May 15, 2024, www.cdc.gov/diabetes/risk-factors/pcos-polycystic-ovary
-syndrome.html.

145 **the average moderately active person may need:** Rajavel Elango, Mohammad A. Humayun, Ronald O. Ball, and Paul B. Pencharz, "Evidence
That Protein Requirements Have Been Significantly Underestimated,"
*Current Opinion in Clinical Nutrition and Metabolic Care* 13, no. 1 (January 2010): 52–57, doi.org/10.1097/mco.0b013e328332f9b7.

### Chapter 6: Simplify Your Relationship with Food

155 **women with ADHD were 3.6 times more likely to have an eating dis-
order:** Alina Rodríguez, Henning Tiemeier, Alan Stein, Joe Murray, and
Terje Falck-Ytter, "Attention-Deficit/Hyperactivity Disorder (ADHD) in
Girls: Clinical Characteristics and Comorbidity," *Social Psychiatry and
Psychiatric Epidemiology* 42 (August 2007): 728–35, doi.org/10.1007
/s00127-007-0227-y.

161 **dull our taste buds:** Carole Bartolotto, "Does Consuming Sugar and Artificial Sweeteners Change Taste Preferences?," *The Permanente Journal*
19, no. 3 (Summer 2015): 81–84, www.ncbi.nlm.nih.gov/pmc/articles
/PMC4500487.

172 **gut microbiome have been linked to attention issues, mood disturbances:** Tae-Hwan Jung, Hyo-Jeong Hwang, and Kyoung-Sik Han, "Correlation of Attention Deficit Hyperactivity Disorder with Gut Microbiota
According to the Dietary Intake of Korean Elementary School Students,"
*PloS One* 17, no. 9 (September 30, 2022): e0275520, www.ncbi.nlm.nih
.gov/pmc/articles/PMC9524712; Megan Clapp, Nadia Aurora, Lindsey
Herrera, Manisha Bhatia, Emily Wilen, and Sarah Wakefield, "Gut Microbiota's Effect on Mental Health: The Gut-Brain Axis," *Clinics and
Practice* 7, no. 4 (September 15, 2017): 987, www.ncbi.nlm.nih.gov/pmc
/articles/PMC5641835.

182 **leading to nutritional deficiencies:** M. Palmery, A. Saraceno, A. Vaiarelli,
and G. Carlomagno, "Oral Contraceptives and Changes in Nutritional
Requirements," *European Review for Medical and Pharmacological
Sciences* 17, no. 13 (July 2013): 1804–13, pubmed.ncbi.nlm.nih.gov
/23852908.

### Chapter 7: Help Your Hormones

186 **influence how we think and act daily:** "Hormones' Role on Our Health,
and Wellness," Weill Cornell Medicine, December 17, 2020, weillcornell
.org/news/hormones'-role-on-our-health-and-wellness.

187 **estrogen plays roles:** "Estrogen," Health Library, Cleveland Clinic,
accessed April 18, 2024, my.clevelandclinic.org/health/body/22353
-estrogen.

188 **It aids in pregnancy:** "Progesterone," Health Library, Cleveland Clinic,

accessed April 18, 2024, my.clevelandclinic.org/health/body/24562
-progesterone.

188 **plays pivotal roles in bone strength:** "Testosterone: What It Is and How
It Affects Your Health," Harvard Health, June 22, 2023, www.health
.harvard.edu/staying-healthy/testosterone--what-it-does-and-doesnt-do.

188 **the hormone responsible for regulating your stress response:** Dani
Blum, "The Truth About the Internet's Favorite Stress Hormone," *The
New York Times,* March 22, 2023, www.nytimes.com/2023/03/22/well
/live/cortisol-stress-hormone.html.

188 **cortisol helps control your metabolism:** "Cortisol," Health Library,
Cleveland Clinic, accessed April 18, 2024, my.clevelandclinic.org/health
/articles/22187-cortisol.

190 **many of us report struggling:** Nathaly Pesantez, "Menstrual Cycle
Phases and ADHD: Why Cycle Syncing Is Essential," *ADDitude,*
May 22, 2024, www.additudemag.com/menstrual-cycle-phases-cycle
-syncing-adhd.

192 **others report experiencing anxiety:** Yael I. Nillni, Donna J. Toufexis,
and Kelly J. Rohan, "Anxiety Sensitivity, the Menstrual Cycle, and Panic
Disorder: A Putative Neuroendocrine and Psychological Interaction,"
*Clinical Psychology Review* 31, no. 7 (November 2011): 1183–91, doi
.org/10.1016/j.cpr.2011.07.006.

192 **intensified ADHD symptoms:** *ADDitude* Editors, "PMS and ADHD:
How the Menstrual Cycle Intensifies Symptoms," *ADDitude,* February 8, 2024, www.additudemag.com/pms-adhd-hormones-menstrual
-cycle.

192 **decline in estrogen:** "Apps Can Help Girls Manage When Hormones
Affect ADHD Symptoms," ADHD Weekly, Children and Adults with
Attention-Deficit/Hyperactivity Disorder (CHADD), March 7, 2024,
chadd.org/adhd-weekly/apps-can-help-girls-manage-when-hormones
-affect-adhd-symptoms.

193 **A sharp rise and sudden drop:** Evangelia Antoniou, Nikolaos Rigas,
Eirini Orovou, Alexandros Papatrechas, and Angeliki Sarella, "ADHD
Symptoms in Females of Childhood, Adolescent, Reproductive and
Menopause Period," *Materia Socio-medica* 33, no. 2 (June 2021):
114–18, www.ncbi.nlm.nih.gov/pmc/articles/PMC8385721.

195 **Women with ADHD often experience more severe symptoms:** Ibid.

195 **Women with PMDD report experiencing:** Divya Prasad, Bianca
Wollenhaupt-Aguiar, Katrina N. Kidd, Taiane de Azevedo Cardoso, and
Benicio N. Frey, "Suicidal Risk in Women with Premenstrual Syndrome
and Premenstrual Dysphoric Disorder: A Systematic Review and Meta-
Analysis," *Journal of Women's Health* 30, no. 12 (December 2021):
1693–707, www.ncbi.nlm.nih.gov/pmc/articles/PMC8721500.

195 **an abnormal sensitivity:** Rebecca A. Clay, "Why Are Some People More

Susceptible to Severe PMS? Psychologists Seek Answers," American
Psychological Association, September 1, 2023, www.apa.org/monitor
/2023/09/emerging-science-severe-pms.

195 **PMDD is:** "What Is PMDD?," International Association for Premenstrual Disorders, accessed May 19, 2024, iapmd.org/about-pmdd.

196 **include adverse childhood experiences:** Liisa Hantsoo and C. Neill
Epperson, "Allopregnanolone in Premenstrual Dysphoric Disorder
(PMDD): Evidence for Dysregulated Sensitivity to GABA-A Receptor
Modulating Neuroactive Steroids Across the Menstrual Cycle," *Neuro-
biology of Stress* 12 (May 2020): 100213, doi.org/10.1016/j.ynstr.2020
.100213.

196 **85 percent of women with PMDD:** Jayashri Kulkarni, Olivia Leyden,
Emorfia Gavrilidis, Caroline Thew, and Elizabeth H. X. Thomas, "The
Prevalence of Early Life Trauma in Premenstrual Dysphoric Disorder
(PMDD)," *Psychiatry Research* 308 (February 2022): 114381, pubmed
.ncbi.nlm.nih.gov/34999294.

199 **higher risk of developing depression:** Cecilia Lundin, Anna Wikman,
Per Wikman, Helena Kopp Kallner, Inger Sundström-Poromaa, and
Charlotte Skoglund, "Hormonal Contraceptive Use and Risk of Depression Among Young Women with Attention-Deficit/Hyperactivity Disorder," *Journal of the American Academy of Child and Adolescent Psychiatry*
62, no. 6 (June 2023): 665–74, pubmed.ncbi.nlm.nih.gov/36332846.

201 **70 to 80 percent of your immune cells:** Selma P. Wiertsema, Jeroen
van Bergenhenegouwen, Johan Garssen, and Leon M. J. Knippels, "The
Interplay Between the Gut Microbiome and the Immune System in the
Context of Infectious Diseases Throughout Life and the Role of Nutrition in Optimizing Treatment Strategies," *Nutrients* 13, no. 3 (March 9,
2021): 886, pubmed.ncbi.nlm.nih.gov/33803407.

202 **estrogen dominance can lead:** Seema Patel, Ahmad Homaei, Akondi
Butchi Raju, and Biswa Ranjan Meher, "Estrogen: The Necessary Evil
for Human Health, and Ways to Tame It," *Biomedicine & Pharmacotherapy* 102 (June 2018): 403–11, pubmed.ncbi.nlm.nih.gov/29573619.

204 **Researchers suggest that human beings:** A. P. Simopoulos, "The Importance of the Ratio of Omega-6/Omega-3 Essential Fatty Acids," *Biomedicine & Pharmacotherapy* 56, no. 8 (October 2002): 365–79, doi
.org/10.1016/s0753-3322(02)00253-6.

206 **lived 34 percent longer:** Victoria Acosta-Rodríguez, Filipa Rijo-Ferreira,
Mariko Izumo, Pin Xu, Mary Wight-Carter, Carla B. Green, and Joseph
S. Takahashi, "Circadian Alignment of Early Onset Caloric Restriction
Promotes Longevity in Male C57BL/6J Mice," *Science* 376, no. 6598
(June 10, 2022): 1192–202, doi.org/10.1126/science.abk0297.

207 **it increases levels of BDNF:** Karin Seidler and Michelle Barrow, "Intermittent Fasting and Cognitive Performance—Targeting BDNF as Poten-

tial Strategy to Optimise Brain Health," *Frontiers in Neuroendocrinology* 65 (April 2022): 100971, doi.org/10.1016/j.yfrne.2021.100971.

207 **supports metabolic health:** Jip Gudden, Alejandro Arias Vasquez, and Mirjam Bloemendaal, "The Effects of Intermittent Fasting on Brain and Cognitive Function," *Nutrients* 13, no. 9 (September 10, 2021): 3166, doi.org/10.3390/nu13093166.

207 **thus improving insulin sensitivity:** Xiaojie Yuan, Jiping Wang, Shuo Yang, Mei Gao, Lingxia Cao, Xumei Li, Dongxu Hong, et al., "Effect of Intermittent Fasting Diet on Glucose and Lipid Metabolism and Insulin Resistance in Patients with Impaired Glucose and Lipid Metabolism: A Systematic Review and Meta-Analysis," *International Journal of Endocrinology* 2022 (March 24, 2022): 1–9, doi.org/10.1155/2022/6999907.

210 **EDCs have been linked:** Saniya Rattan, Changqing Zhou, Catheryne Chiang, Sharada Mahalingam, Emily Brehm, and Jodi A. Flaws, "Exposure to Endocrine Disruptors During Adulthood: Consequences for Female Fertility," *Journal of Endocrinology* 233, no. 3 (June 2017): R109–29, doi.org/10.1530/joe-17-0023.

210 **such as endometriosis, PCOS, irregular periods, early puberty, cancer, and infertility, as well as neurological and learning disabilities:** Livia Interdonato, Rosalba Siracusa, Roberta Fusco, Salvatore Cuzzocrea, and Rosanna Di Paola, "Endocrine Disruptor Compounds in Environment: Focus on Women's Reproductive Health and Endometriosis," *International Journal of Molecular Sciences* 24, no. 6 (March 16, 2023): 5682, doi.org/10.3390/ijms24065682; Tinkara Srnovršnik, Irma Virant-Klun, and Bojana Pinter, "Polycystic Ovary Syndrome and Endocrine Disruptors (Bisphenols, Parabens, and Triclosan)—a Systematic Review," *Life* 13, no. 1 (January 4, 2023): 138, doi.org/10.3390/life13010138; Saquib Hassan, Aswin Thacharodi, Anshu Priya, R. Meenatchi, Thanushree A. Hegde, Thangamani R, H. T. Nguyen, et al., "Endocrine Disruptors: Unravelling the Link Between Chemical Exposure and Women's Reproductive Health," *Environmental Research* 241 (January 15, 2024): 117385, doi.org/10.1016/j.envres.2023.117385; Anastasios Papadimitriou and Dimitrios Papadimitriou, "Endocrine-Disrupting Chemicals and Early Puberty in Girls," *Children* 8, no. 6 (June 10, 2021): 492, doi.org/10.3390/children8060492; R. Modica, E. Benevento, and A. Colao, "Endocrine-Disrupting Chemicals (EDCs) and Cancer: New Perspectives on an Old Relationship," *Journal of Endocrinological Investigation* 46, no. 4 (December 16, 2022): 667–77, doi.org/10.1007/s40618-022-01983-4; Joseph Pizzorno, "Environmental Toxins and Infertility," *Integrative Medicine* 17, no. 2 (April 2018), 8–11, https://www.ncbi.nlm.nih.gov/pmc/articles/PMC6396757; Abhinandan Ghosh, Adrija Tripathy, and Debidas Ghosh, "Impact of Endocrine Disrupting Chemicals (EDCs) on Reproductive Health of Human," *Proceedings of*

*the Zoological Society* 75, no. 1 (March 6, 2022): 16–30, doi.org/10.1007 /s12595-021-00412-3; Małgorzata Kajta and Anna K. Wójtowicz, "Impact of Endocrine-Disrupting Chemicals on Neural Development and the Onset of Neurological Disorders," *Pharmacological Reports* 65, no. 6 (November–December 2013): 1632–39, doi.org/10.1016/s1734 -1140(13)71524-x; "Impact of EDCs on Neurological and Behavioral Systems," Endocrine Society, accessed May 18, 2024, www.endocrine .org/topics/edc/what-edcs-are/common-edcs/neurological.

210 **neurotransmitters like dopamine and norepinephrine:** Thaddeus T. Schug, Ashley M. Blawas, Kimberly Gray, Jerrold J. Heindel, and Cindy P. Lawler, "Elucidating the Links Between Endocrine Disruptors and Neurodevelopment," *Endocrinology* 156, no. 6 (June 2015): 1941–51, www.ncbi.nlm.nih.gov/pmc/articles/PMC5393340.

211 **BPA, found primarily in plastics:** Ibid.

211 **increased toxic burden:** Chris Gennings, Rhonda Ellis, and Joseph K. Ritter, "Linking Empirical Estimates of Body Burden of Environmental Chemicals and Wellness Using NHANES Data," *Environment International* 39, no. 1 (February 2012): 56–65, doi.org/10.1016/j.envint.2011 .09.002.

211 **"Endocrine-disrupting chemicals present in our food":** "Endocrine-Disrupting Chemicals May Raise Risk of Cognitive Disorders in Future Generations," *ScienceDaily,* June 15, 2023, www.sciencedaily.com /releases/2023/06/230615183239.htm.

211 **One 2020 study found that exposure to common phthalates:** "Phthalates," Breast Cancer Prevention Partners, 2021, www.bcpp.org/resource /phthalates.

211 **"associated with behaviors characteristic of ADHD":** Jessica R. Shoaff, Brent Coull, Jennifer Weuve, David C. Bellinger, Antonia M. Calafat, Susan L. Schantz, and Susan A. Korrick, "Association of Exposure to Endocrine-Disrupting Chemicals During Adolescence with Attention-Deficit/Hyperactivity Disorder-Related Behaviors," *JAMA Network Open* 3, no. 8 (August 3, 2020): e2015041, pubmed.ncbi.nlm.nih .gov/32857150.

211 **Another study, from 2018, found that moms:** Stephanie M. Engel, Gro D. Villanger, Rachel C. Nethery, Cathrine Thomsen, Amrit K. Sakhi, Samantha S. M. Drover, Jane A. Hoppin, et al., "Prenatal Phthalates, Maternal Thyroid Function, and Risk of Attention-Deficit Hyperactivity Disorder in the Norwegian Mother and Child Cohort," *Environmental Health Perspectives* 126, no. 5 (May 10, 2018), ehp.niehs.nih.gov/doi /10.1289/EHP2358.

211 **increased risk of future generations of their families:** Marianthi-Anna Kioumourtzoglou, Brent A. Coull, Éilis J. O'Reilly, Alberto Ascherio, and Marc G. Weisskopf, "Association of Exposure to Diethylstilbestrol During Pregnancy with Multigenerational Neurodevelopmental Deficits,"

*JAMA Pediatrics* 172, no. 7 (July 1, 2018): 670–77, doi.org/10.1001
/jamapediatrics.2018.0727.nih.gov/29799929.

212 **36 percent more likely to have ADHD:** "Pregnancy Drug DES Linked
to ADHD in Users' Grandchildren," Columbia University Mailman
School of Public Health, May 22, 2018, www.publichealth.columbia
.edu/news/pregnancy-drug-des-linked-adhd-users-grandchildren.

212 **"multigenerational neurodevelopmental deficits":** Marianthi-Anna
Kioumourtzoglou, Brent A. Coull, Éilis J. O'Reilly, Alberto Ascherio, and
Marc G. Weisskopf, "Association of Exposure to Diethylstilbestrol Dur-
ing Pregnancy with Multigenerational Neurodevelopmental Deficits,"
*JAMA Pediatrics* 172, no. 7 (July 1, 2018): 670–77, doi.org/10.1001
/jamapediatrics.2018.0727.

212 **According to the Environmental Working Group:** "Why Skin Deep®?,"
EWG's Skin Deep, accessed May 19, 2024, www.ewg.org/skindeep
/learn_more/why-skin-deep.

215 **Cleaning products, detergents:** Inhye Lee and Kyunghee Ji, "Identifica-
tion of Combinations of Endocrine Disrupting Chemicals in Household
Chemical Products That Require Mixture Toxicity Testing," *Ecotoxicol-
ogy and Environmental Safety* 240 (July 15, 2022): 113677, doi.org
/10.1016/j.ecoenv.2022.113677.

217 **cancer-related cell behaviors:** Shanaz H. Dairkee, Dan H. Moore,
M. Gloria Luciani, Nicole Anderle, Roy Gerona, Karina Ky, Saman-
tha M. Torres, et al., "Reduction of Daily-Use Parabens and Phthalates
Reverses Accumulation of Cancer-Associated Phenotypes Within
Disease-Free Breast Tissue of Study Subjects," *Chemosphere* 322 (May
2023): 138014, doi.org/10.1016/j.chemosphere.2023.138014.

218 **increasing the risk of autoimmune diseases:** Ljudmila Stojanovich and
Dragomir Marisavljevich, "Stress as a Trigger of Autoimmune Disease,"
*Autoimmunity Reviews* 7, no. 3 (January 2008): 209–13, doi.org/10.1016
/j.autrev.2007.11.007.

**Chapter 8: Regulate Your Nervous System and Reconnect**

223 **a number of studies have found:** Corey E. Pilver, Becca R. Levy, Daniel J. Libby, and Rani A. Desai, "Posttraumatic Stress Disorder and
Trauma Characteristics Are Correlates of Premenstrual Dysphoric Disor-
der," *Archives of Women's Mental Health* 14, no. 5 (July 23, 2011):
383–93, doi.org/10.1007/s00737-011-0232-4; Mikael Landén, Bertil
Wennerblom, Hans Tygesen, Kjell Modigh, Karin Sörvik, Christina
Ysander, Agneta Ekman, et al., "Heart Rate Variability in Premenstrual
Dysphoric Disorder," *Psychoneuroendocrinology* 29, no. 6 (July 2004):
733–40, doi.org/10.1016/s0306-4530(03)00117-3; Tamaki Matsumoto,
Takahisa Ushiroyama, Tetsuya Kimura, Tatsuya Hayashi, and Toshio
Moritani, "Altered Autonomic Nervous System Activity as a Potential
Etiological Factor of Premenstrual Syndrome and Premenstrual Dys-

phoric Disorder," *BioPsychoSocial Medicine* 1, no. 1 (2007): 24, doi
.org/10.1186/1751-0759-1-24.

223 **"rooted in multi-generational family stress":** "Dr. Gabor Maté," n.d.,
drgabormate.com/adhd.

228 **Low vagal tone:** Megan Anna Neff, "The Autistic and ADHD Nervous
System," Neurodivergent Insights, neurodivergentinsights.com/blog
/autistic-adhd-nervous-system.

228 **Spoiler: Those of us with ADHD:** "Heart Rate Variability (HRV) in
ADHD," ADxS.org, accessed September 27, 2023, www.adxs.org/en
/page/96/heart-rate-variability-hrv-in-adhd.

230 **Emerging evidence suggests:** Rachel Yehuda and Amy Lehrner, "Inter-
generational Transmission of Trauma Effects: Putative Role of Epigenetic Mechanisms," *World Psychiatry* 17, no. 3 (September 7, 2018):
243–57, doi.org/10.1002/wps.20568.

232 **activate mast cells (a type of white blood cell) to release histamines:**
Ann L. Baldwin, "Mast Cell Activation by Stress," in *Mast Cells: Methods
and Protocols,* ed. Guha Krishnaswamy and David S. Chi (Totowa, NJ:
Humana Press, 2006), 349–60, doi.org/10.1385/1-59259-967-2:349.

232 **if one has a regulated nervous system:** Sarah E. Johnstone and Ste-
phen B. Baylin, "Stress and the Epigenetic Landscape: A Link to the
Pathobiology of Human Diseases?," *Nature Reviews Genetics* 11, no. 11
(October 5, 2010): 806–12, doi.org/10.1038/nrg2881.

257 **Many sleep experts emphasize:** Angus S. Fisk, Shu K. E. Tam, Lau-
rence A. Brown, Vladyslav V. Vyazovskiy, David M. Bannerman, and Stu-
art N. Peirson, "Light and Cognition: Roles for Circadian Rhythms,
Sleep, and Arousal," *Frontiers in Neurology* 9 (February 8, 2018), doi
.org/10.3389/fneur.2018.00056.

258 **natural light is a cue:** Christine Blume, Corrado Garbazza, and Manuel
Spitschan, "Effects of Light on Human Circadian Rhythms, Sleep and
Mood," *Somnologie* 23, no. 3 (August 20, 2019): 147–56, doi.org/10
.1007/s11818-019-00215-x.

259 **restorative form of deep sleep:** Danielle Pacheco and Abhinav Singh,
"How Much Deep Sleep Do You Need?," Sleep Foundation, March 22,
2024, www.sleepfoundation.org/stages-of-sleep/deep-sleep; "Sleep
Physiology," in *Sleep Disorders and Sleep Deprivation: An Unmet Public
Health Problem,* ed. Harvey R. Colten and Bruce M. Altevogt (Washington, DC: National Academies Press, 2006), www.ncbi.nlm.nih.gov
/books/NBK19956.

259 **the glymphatic system:** Yo-El S. Ju, Sharon J. Ooms, Courtney Sutphen,
Shannon L. Macauley, Margaret A. Zangrilli, Gina Jerome, Anne M.
Fagan, et al., "Slow Wave Sleep Disruption Increases Cerebrospinal
Fluid Amyloid-β Levels," *Brain* 140, no. 8 (August 2017): 2104–11, doi
.org/10.1093/brain/awx148.

260 **when our melatonin level peaks:** Jean-Philippe Chaput, Caroline Dutil, Ryan Featherstone, Robert Ross, Lora Giangregorio, Travis J. Saunders, Ian Janssen, et al., "Sleep Timing, Sleep Consistency, and Health in Adults: A Systematic Review," *Applied Physiology, Nutrition, and Metabolism* 45, no. 10 (Suppl. 2) (October 2020), doi.org/10.1139/apnm-2020 -0032.

266 **effective in helping:** Clotilde Guidetti, Patrizia Brogna, Daniela Pia Rosaria Chieffo, Ida Turrini, Valentina Arcangeli, Azzurra Rausa, Maddalena Bianchetti, et al., "Eye Movement Desensitization and Reprocessing (EMDR) as a Possible Evidence-Based Rehabilitation Treatment Option for a Patient with ADHD and History of Adverse Childhood Experiences: A Case Report Study," *Journal of Personalized Medicine* 13, no. 2 (January 23, 2023): 200, doi.org/10.3390/jpm13020200; "Is EMDR Effective for Treating ADHD?," PESI, accessed May 20, 2024, www.pesi.com/blog/details/2105/is-emdr-effective-for-treating-adhd.

271 **"virtues our culture rewards":** Maytal Eyal, "Self-Silencing Is Making Women Sick," *TIME*, October 3, 2023, time.com/6319549/silencing -women-sick-essay.

271 **a condition associated with nervous system dysregulation:** Chiara Bellocchi, Angelica Carandina, Beatrice Montinaro, Elena Targetti, Ludovico Furlan, Gabriel Dias Rodrigues, Eleonora Tobaldini, et al., "The Interplay Between Autonomic Nervous System and Inflammation Across Systemic Autoimmune Diseases," *International Journal of Molecular Sciences* 23, no. 5 (February 23, 2022): 2449, doi.org/10.3390 /ijms23052449.

271 **"Hyperfunctioning on top of hidden distress":** Gabor Maté, *The Myth of Normal: Trauma, Illness, and Healing in a Toxic Culture* (London: Random House UK, 2023).

272 **"Anger does not require hostile acting out":** Gabor Maté, *When the Body Says No: Exploring the Stress-Disease Connection* (Hoboken, NJ: Wiley, 2011).

**Appendix: Supplements**

277 **how the body reacts to stress:** S. B. Sartori, N. Whittle, A. Hetzenauer, and N. Singewald, "Magnesium Deficiency Induces Anxiety and HPA Axis Dysregulation: Modulation by Therapeutic Drug Treatment," *Neuropharmacology* 62, no. 1 (January 2012): 304–12, doi.org/10.1016/j .neuropharm.2011.07.027.

277 **increase the activity of GABA:** *Magnesium in the Central Nervous System,* Chapter 7, ed. Robert Vink and Mihai Nechifor (Adelaide, Australia: University of Adelaide Press, 2011).

277 **lower GABA levels or impaired GABA receptor function:** Anthony S. Ferranti, Deborah J. Luessen, and Colleen M. Niswender, "Novel Phar-

macological Targets for GABAergic Dysfunction in ADHD," *Neuropharmacology* 249 (May 2024): 109897, doi.org/10.1016/j.neuropharm .2024.109897.

278 **anemia, depression, anxiety, and miscarriage:** Ashley Marcin, "MTHFR Gene Mutation," Healthline, June 3, 2024, www.healthline .com/health/mthfr-gene; Shailesh Jha, Pankaj Kumar, Rajesh Kumar, and Aparna Das, "Effectiveness of Add-On L-Methylfolate Therapy in a Complex Psychiatric Illness with MTHFR C677 T Genetic Polymorphism," *Asian Journal of Psychiatry* 22 (August 2016): 74–75, doi .org/10.1016/j.ajp.2016.05.007.

278 **linked to more than sixty conditions:** Lin Wan, Yuhong Li, Zhengrong Zhang, Zuoli Sun, Yi He, and Rena Li, "Methylenetetrahydrofolate Reductase and Psychiatric Diseases," *Translational Psychiatry* 8, no. 1 (November 5, 2018), doi.org/10.1038/s41398-018-0276-6.

278 **up to 40 percent of the population:** Ashley Marcin, "MTHFR Gene Mutation," Healthline, June 3, 2024, www.healthline.com/health /mthfr-gene.

279 **In a study comparing saffron to fluoxetine:** Fatemeh Rajabi, Marjan Rahimi, Mohammad Reza Sharbafchizadeh, and Mohammad Javad Tarrahi, "Saffron for the Management of Premenstrual Dysphoric Disorder: A Randomized Controlled Trial," *Advanced Biomedical Research* 9, no. 1 (2020): 60, doi.org/10.4103/abr.abr_49_20.

279 **A study done on adolescents:** Sara Baziar, Ali Aqamolaei, Ebrahim Khadem, Seyyed Hosein Mortazavi, Sina Naderi, Erfan Sahebolzamani, Amirhosein Mortezaei, et al., "*Crocus sativus* L. Versus Methylphenidate in Treatment of Children with Attention-Deficit/Hyperactivity Disorder: A Randomized, Double-Blind Pilot Study," *Journal of Child and Adolescent Psychopharmacology* 29, no. 3 (April 3, 2019): 205–12, doi.org /10.1089/cap.2018.0146.

279 **Saffron's neuroprotective properties:** "Can Saffron Help with ADHD?," *Medical News Today,* June 28, 2023, www.medicalnewstoday .com/articles/saffron-adhd.

279 **Its use during pregnancy:** Jennifer Larson, "Is Saffron (Kesar) Safe During Pregnancy?," Healthline, January 28, 2021, www.healthline.com /health/pregnancy/saffron-during-pregnancy.

279 **even depressed:** Sue Penckofer, Joanne Kouba, Mary Byrn, and Carol Estwing Ferrans, "Vitamin D and Depression: Where Is All the Sunshine?," *Issues in Mental Health Nursing* 31, no. 6 (May 7, 2010): 385–93, doi.org/10.3109/01612840903437657.

279 **children with ADHD have lower vitamin D levels:** Armon Massoodi, Sakineh Javadian Koutanaei, Zahra Faraz, Zahra Geraili, and Seyedeh Maryam Zavarmousavi, "Comparison of Serum Vitamin D Levels Between Healthy and ADHD Children," *Caspian Journal of Internal Medicine* 14, no. 4 (Fall 2023): 681–86, doi.org/10.22088/cjim.14.4.68.

280 **recommended for PMS:** Dezső Csupor, Tamás Lantos, Péter Hegyi, Ria
    Benkő, Réka Viola, Zoltán Gyöngyi, Péter Csécsei, et al., "*Vitex agnus-
    castus* in Premenstrual Syndrome: A Meta-Analysis of Double-Blind Ran-
    domised Controlled Trials," *Complementary Therapies in Medicine* 47
    (December 2019): 102190, doi.org/10.1016/j.ctim.2019.08.024.
280 **great for liver health:** Ted George O. Achufusi, Mark V. Pellegrini, and
    Raj K. Patel, "Milk Thistle," StatPearls, 2024, www.ncbi.nlm.nih.gov
    /books/NBK541075.
280 **use during pregnancy or breastfeeding:** Jean-Jacques Dugoua, Dugald
    Seely, Daniel Perri, Gideon Koren, and Edward Mills, "Safety and Effi-
    cacy of Chastetree (*Vitex agnus-castus*) During Pregnancy and Lactation,"
    *Canadian Journal of Clinical Pharmacology* 15, no. 1 (Winter 2008):
    e74–79, pubmed.ncbi.nlm.nih.gov/18204102.

# Index

LISA DEE is an Irish health and fitness coach based in London with more than a decade's worth of experience. She has guided thousands of women through body and mindset transformations on the gym floor and online. After being diagnosed with ADHD as an adult, Dee created Healthy Happy ADHD, an online platform to help women with ADHD to build healthy habits and improve their self-image.

**ABOUT THE TYPE**

This book was set in Fairfield, the first typeface from the hand of the distinguished American artist and engraver Rudolph Ruzicka (1883–1978). Ruzicka was born in Bohemia (in the present-day Czech Republic) and came to America in 1894. He set up his own shop, devoted to wood engraving and printing, in New York in 1913 after a varied career working as a wood engraver, in photoengraving and banknote printing plants, and as an art director and freelance artist. He designed and illustrated many books, and was the creator of a considerable list of individual prints—wood engravings, line engravings on copper, and aquatints.